Obs and Gynae

PG Focus Series

Caesarean Birth

Past, Present and Optimizing the Future

Obs and Gynae PG Focus Series

Caesarean Birth

Past, Present and Optimizing the Future

Editors

Niranjan Chavan

MD FICOG FCPS DGO DFP MICOG DICOG Diploma in Endoscopy (USA)
Professor and Unit Chief
Department of Obstetrics and Gynaecology
Lokmanya Tilak Medical College and General Hospital
Mumbai, Maharashtra, India

Komal N Chavan

MD DNB MNAMS FCPS DGO FICOG and Diploma in Reproductive Medicine (UK-SH Germany)
Senior Consultant and Unit Chief
Department of Obstetrics and Gynaecology
VN Desai Hospital
Mumbai, Maharashtra, India

Co-Editors

Madhura Mandlik

MBBS MS (Obs/Gynae)
Senior Resident
Department of Obstetrics and Gynaecology
Lokmanya Tilak Medical College and General Hospital
Mumbai, Maharashtra, India

Shruti Rane

MBBS
Junior Resident 3
Department of Obstetrics and Gynaecology
Lokmanya Tilak Medical College and General Hospital
Mumbai, Maharashtra, India

JAYPEE

JAYPEE BROTHERS MEDICAL PUBLISHERS

The Health Sciences Publisher

New Delhi | London

Jaypee Brothers Medical Publishers (P) Ltd

Headquarters

Jaypee Brothers Medical Publishers (P) Ltd
EMCA House, 23/23-B
Ansari Road, Daryaganj
New Delhi 110 002, India
Landline: +91-11-23272143, +91-11-23272703
+91-11-23282021, +91-11-23245672
Email: jaypee@jaypeebrothers.com

Corporate Office

Jaypee Brothers Medical Publishers (P) Ltd
4838/24, Ansari Road, Daryaganj
New Delhi 110 002, India
Phone: +91-11-43574357
Fax: +91-11-43574314
Email: jaypee@jaypeebrothers.com

Overseas Office

JP Medical Ltd.
83, Victoria Street, London
SW1H 0HW (UK)
Phone: +44 20 3170 8910
Fax: +44 (0)20 3008 6180
Email: info@jpmedpub.com

Website: www.jaypeebrothers.com
Website: www.jaypeedigital.com

Obs and Gynae PG Focus Series: Caesarean Birth: Past, Present and Optimizing the Future

First Edition: **2025**

ISBN: 978-93-6616-674-2

Printed in India

Preface

Caesarean birth, once a rare and often life-saving procedure, has become a cornerstone of modern obstetric practice. Its evolution over the years has reshaped the landscape of childbirth, offering a solution to various complications that may arise during labor, such as fetal distress, maternal health concerns, and abnormal presentations. Today, caesarean sections account for a significant proportion of deliveries worldwide, providing patients with the benefits of a safer childbirth experience in certain clinical scenarios. For obstetricians, mastering the indications, technique, and post-operative care of caesarean births is essential to ensuring the best outcomes for both mother and child.

This manual is designed to serve as a comprehensive guide for both novice and experienced practitioners seeking to expand their knowledge and skills in caesarean birth. From the historical roots and evolution of caesarean procedures to the current best practices, it offers a structured approach to understanding the technique, along with practical advice on managing complications and optimizing outcomes. Whether performing an elective or emergency caesarean section, the goal remains constant: to provide the safest and most effective care for both the mother and her baby.

The manual highlights essential topics, including the indications for caesarean birth, surgical techniques, anesthesia considerations, and post-operative care.

And most importantly this book emphasizes the use of Sion Model devised by Dr Niranjan Chavan which has improved vaginal birth rates since July 2023.

It also delves into important discussions on minimizing complications, improving patient outcomes, and addressing the growing concern of unnecessary caesarean sections in modern obstetrics, enhanced recovery protocols, and strategies for reducing the caesarean section rate while ensuring patient safety.

We hope this manual serves as an indispensable resource in your practice, aiding you in providing the highest standard of care, promoting informed decision-making, and optimizing surgical outcomes for your patients.

Editors
Niranjan Chavan
Komal N Chavan

Co-Editors
Madhura Mandlik
Shruti Rane

Acknowledgments

With immense gratitude, we express our sincere thanks to all those who contributed to the completion of *Caesarean Birth: Past, Present and Optimizing the Future*. This endeavor would not have been possible without the encouragement and support of many individuals.

We extend our deepest thanks to all the authors and co-authors for sharing their expertise and their commitment to producing a resource of the highest standards.

Our heartfelt appreciation goes to our mentors and colleagues, whose valuable insights and guidance inspired the structure and content of this book. Their expertise and shared experiences have significantly enriched its scope.

To our families and friends: Your unwavering support, patience, and encouragement during the demanding phases of this project have been our greatest strength.

We would also like to acknowledge Dr Niranjan Chavan unit members—Dr Deepali (Associate Professor), Dr Swara (Assistant Professor), Dr Vishwaja (Assistant Professor), and all the Junior Residents—Dr Darshana Ajmera, Dr Radhika Bhutada, Dr Monika Dhauchak, Dr Juili Tadkar, and Dr Rutuja Mohite for their dedication, time, and hard work. Their efforts, in addition to managing their hectic schedules, were instrumental in bringing this book to life.

We especially appreciate the constant support and encouragement of Shri Jitendar P Vij (Group Chairman) and Mr Ankit Vij (Managing Director) of M/s Jaypee Brothers Medical Publishers (P) Ltd, New Delhi, India, in publishing the book and their associates, particularly Ms Chetna Malhotra (Senior Director—Professional Publishing, Marketing, and Business Development), Ms Kritika Dua (Senior Commissiong Editor), Mr Pragati Singh and Mr Priyansh Saxena (Development Editors), who have been prompt, efficient, and most helpful.

Lastly, to the readers and practitioners of obstetrics and gynaecology, we hope this book serves as a valuable resource, contributing to the betterment of patient care and surgical practice.

Thank you all for being a part of this journey.

Contents

CHAPTER 1

Introduction

A caesarean section is the surgical delivery of a baby, whether alive or deceased, through an incision in the abdomen and uterus after the point of viability. The term "caesarean" comes from the Latin word "caedare," which means "to cut." Thanks to advancements like antibiotics, improved anesthesia, and blood transfusions, this operation has become increasingly common. However, it's crucial to ensure that C-sections are performed for legitimate medical reasons, rather than due to a lack of obstetric skills compared to earlier practices. While modern technology has made the procedure safer, careful evaluation and adherence to guidelines are essential to prioritize the health of both the mother and the baby. Overusing C-sections can introduce unnecessary risks, highlighting the need for skilled obstetric care and thoughtful decision-making before opting for surgical delivery.

While the procedure is considerably safer now, the criteria for performing caesarean sections and their rates are still under scrutiny, as the complication rates remain significantly higher than those associated with vaginal delivery.

HISTORY

The practice of caesarean section dates back to ancient times, specifically during the reign of Numa Pompilius in Rome (715–672 BC). It was primarily performed in the hope of delivering a living child when the mother was deceased or close to death, with little regard for the mother's survival. The term "caesarean section" was first coined by James Guillimeau and the earliest documented caesarean birth occurred in 1020 AD.[1] In those early days, if the mother was still alive, some form of anesthesia—typically alcohol—was used. The advent of anesthetics in the nineteenth century allowed for the procedure to be taken more seriously.

Caesarean sections have been recorded in both Western and non-Western histories. In Greek mythology, it is said that Asclepius was delivered from his mother's abdomen by Apollo. Similarly, Indian history from the Mauryan Empire mentions an instance involving Chanakya, the advisor to King Chandragupta. According to the story, when the king's wife was accidentally poisoned while pregnant with Bindusara, Chandragupta delivered the baby by opening her abdomen.[1]

A more recent documented case of a caesarean section dates back to the 1580s in Siegershausen, Switzerland. The origin of the term "caesarean" remains unclear. It is likely derived from the *Lex Regia* (Royal Law) established by Roman King Numa Pompilius in 715 BC. This law mandated that if a pregnant woman died before giving birth, the baby had to be delivered through the abdomen before burial. The practice persisted under the rule of the Caesars, during which it became known as the *Lex Caesarea*

Despite the advancements in technique, the death rate from caesarean sections remained as high as 75% until 1878, when Murdoch Cameron in Glasgow successfully performed eight caesarean deliveries without any maternal fatalities. Prior to this, the main causes of maternal death were shock, sepsis, and hemorrhage, largely due to the practice of leaving the uterus unsutured after surgery. In 1876, the Italian obstetrician Porro developed a technique involving the amputation of the uterus at the internal os and fixation of the cervical stumps within the abdominal incision. This method significantly improved mortality rates by eliminating the risk of ongoing intraperitoneal bleeding. In 1882, German gynaecologist, Max Sanger, introduced the classical caesarean technique and advocated for suturing the uterine incision with gut sutures, which greatly reduced the risk of hemorrhage and the need for caesarean hysterectomy. He is often regarded as the father of modern caesarean section. The success of suturing the uterine wound rekindled interest in the classical operation during the late 19th century. Interestingly, the history of lower-segment caesarean sections dates back further than expected, with Osiander performing a procedure of this type in 1805.

In 1821, Ritgen made a failed attempt at an extraperitoneal caesarean section, resulting in the mother's death despite the baby being born alive. At the beginning of the twentieth century, in 1907, Frank developed a type of extraperitoneal procedure for cases involving an infected uterus. He sutured

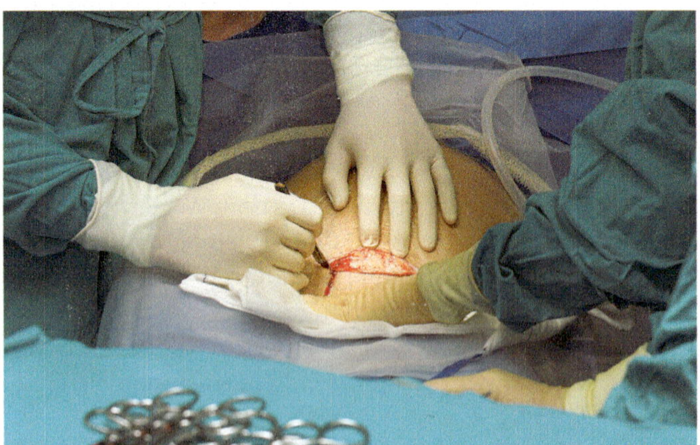

Fig. 1: Pfannenstiel incision during caesarean section.

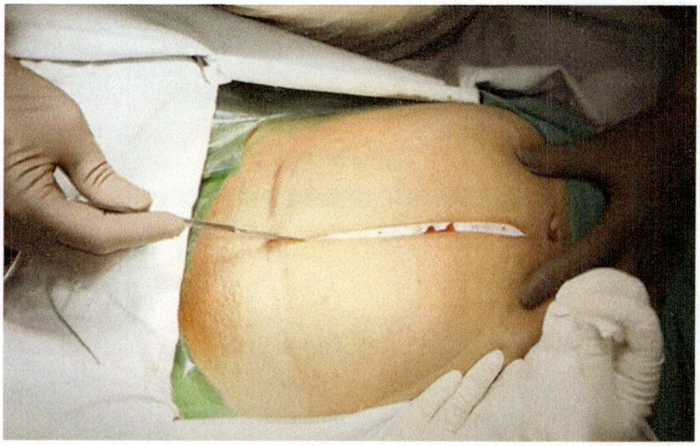

Fig. 2: Vertical incision during caesarean section.

the upper edge of the parietal peritoneum to the visceral peritoneum and made a transverse incision in the lower segment of the uterus. In 1912, Kronig modified this technique, arguing against the extraperitoneal approach and introducing the transperitoneal lower segment caesarean section instead. It was Munro Kerr in 1926 who first described the lower segment transverse uterine incision and helped popularize the procedure.[2] **Figure 1** showing Pfannenstiel incision during caesarean section. **Figure 2** showing vertical incision during caesarean section.

REFERENCES

1. Chavan N. Caesarean Delivery. In: Sharma A (Ed). Labour Room Emergencies. Singapore: Springer Singapore; 2020. pp. 297-303. A
2. Kerr JMM. The technic of cesarean section, with special reference to the lower uterine segment incision. Am J Obstet Gynecol. 1926;12(5):729-34.

CHAPTER 2

Classification

INTRODUCTION

Several classifications have been proposed to analyze caesarean section rates among different risk groups. The goal of categorizing women is to identify those for whom effective strategies, such as changes in labor management protocols, can help optimize caesarean section rates. Robson's classification **(Table 1)** is widely regarded as the most effective for auditing caesarean section rates in both low-risk and high-risk groups.

CLASSIFICATION BASED ON URGENCY

- *Category 1:* Immediate threat to the life of the woman or fetus (for example, suspected uterine rupture, major placental abruption, cord

TABLE 1: Robson's classification for caesarean sections.[1]

Group	*Obstetric population*
1	Nulliparous, single cephalic pregnancy, at least 37 weeks' gestation, spontaneous labor
2	Nulliparous, single cephalic pregnancy, at least 37 weeks' gestation, with either induced labor or a caesarean section prior to the onset of spontaneous labor
3	Multiparous, no previous caesarean section, single cephalic pregnancy, at least 37 weeks' gestation, spontaneous labor
4	Multiparous, no previous caesarean section, single cephalic pregnancy, at least 37 weeks' gestation, with either induced labor or a caesarean section prior to the onset of spontaneous labor
5	Previous caesarean section, single cephalic pregnancy, at least 37 weeks' gestation
6	Nulliparous, single breech pregnancy, with previous caesarean section
7	Multiparous, single breech pregnancy, including previous caesarean section
8	Multiparous, including previous caesarean section
9	Single pregnancy with transverse or oblique lie, including previous caesarean section
10	Single cephalic pregnancy, 36 weeks' gestation or less, including previous caesarean section

prolapse, fetal hypoxia, or persistent fetal bradycardia). Baby should be delivered within 30 minutes.

- *Category 2:* Maternal or fetal compromise which is not immediately life-threatening. Baby should be delivered within 75 minutes.
- *Category 3:* No maternal or fetal compromise but needs early birth.
- *Category 4:* Birth timed to suit woman or healthcare provider.

INCIDENCE

The incidence of caesarean sections is increasing globally. In addition to the rise in medically necessary procedures due to improved access to hospital care, there has been a notable uptick in caesarean sections performed for less accepted medical reasons, such as perceived safety for the baby, reduced pelvic floor trauma, avoidance of labor pains, and convenience. The World Health Organization has stated that there is no justification for any region to have a caesarean section rate exceeding 10–15%. A recent systematic review found that caesarean rates above 10% do not correlate with lower maternal and newborn mortality rates. However, many affluent societies have surpassed these figures, raising concerns within public health.

Caesarean section rates are rising in both developed and developing countries. A global report from 2018 indicated that the worldwide caesarean rate nearly doubled, increasing from 12% in 2000 to 21% in 2015.[2] During this same period, North America's rates rose from 24 to 32%, while South Asia's rates climbed from 7.2 to 18%. In low- and middle-income countries, disparities were evident based on women's financial status; countries with a national average of 26% had a caesarean rate of 14.8% among the poorest women compared to 39.4% in the wealthiest quintile.

A study conducted in Sydney, Australia, examined trends in the indications for caesarean sections over three decades. The rate of caesarean births rose from 18.7% between 1989 and 1994 to 30.4% from 2010 to 2016, with the most significant increases observed in Robson groups 6, 7, and 8 (term breech and multiple pregnancies). In a Central American country, a general hospital reported a caesarean section rate of 59.8%, with 53.9% of these procedures occurring in low-risk groups (Robson 1–4) and 22% being repeat caesareans. This data suggests that to reduce overall caesarean rates, efforts should concentrate on low-risk women, where procedures are often performed for reasons such as failure to progress, presumed fetal distress, and abnormal cardiotocograph readings. Additionally, there is considerable variability in caesarean rates between public and private institutions, with some private facilities in Brazil reporting rates as high as 70%.

REFERENCES

1. Vogel JP, Betrán AP, Vindevoghel N, Souza JP, Torloni MR, Zhang J, et al. Use of the Robson classification to assess caesarean section trends in 21 countries: a secondary analysis of two WHO multicountry surveys. Lancet Glob Health. 2015;3(5):e260-70.
2. Khatamee M. Historical perspective "Rostam" is born: how? By Cesarean section (940-1020 ?). ACOG Clin Rev. 2000;5(2):12.

3

CHAPTER

Maternal Morbidity and Mortality

INTRODUCTION

In 1885, the operative mortality rate for caesarean births was 85% in Great Britain and Ireland, and it rose to 92% in New York by 1887. By the early 20th century, this rate had decreased to <10%, even though the classical operation was predominantly performed during that time. In high-resource settings today, maternal mortality is rare; however, the risk of death following a caesarean section remains three times higher than that of vaginal birth. Data from the Confidential Enquiry into Maternal Deaths in the Netherlands from 1999 to 2013 indicated a mortality risk of 21.9 per 100,000 caesarean sections compared to 3.8 deaths per 100,000 vaginal births. In contrast, low- and middle-income countries report a maternal mortality rate of 7.6 per 1,000, with the highest rates occurring in sub-Saharan Africa (10.9 per 1,000). Notably, a quarter of all maternal deaths in these regions involved women who had undergone a caesarean section. The maternal mortality rate associated with caesarean deliveries is approximately 2.2 per 100,000, significantly higher than the rate for vaginal deliveries, which is about 0.2 per 100,000.[1,2]

In 1885, the operative mortality rate for caesarean births was 85% in Great Britain and Ireland, rising to 92% in New York by 1887. By the early 20th century, this rate had dropped to below 10%, despite the continued prevalence of the classical operation during that era. Today, maternal mortality is rare in high-resource settings, yet the risk of death following a caesarean section is still three times higher than that associated with vaginal delivery. Women who had caesarean deliveries also faced increased risks of postpartum cardiac arrest, wound hematoma, major puerperal infections, anesthetic complications, venous thromboembolism (VTE), and hemorrhage requiring hysterectomy compared to those who delivered vaginally.[3]

In addition to immediate morbidity and mortality, caesarean births are linked to significant long-term health issues. They elevate the risk of future infertility, placental abnormalities, uterine rupture, and stillbirth. The likelihood of conditions such as placenta previa, placenta accreta, and placental abruption also rises in subsequent pregnancies. Specifically, the risk of placenta accreta increases from 3% after the first caesarean to 11% after the second, 40% after the third, and 60% after the fourth caesarean section. Additionally, women with a history of caesarean delivery face a higher risk of complications if they require a hysterectomy later in life.

FETAL RISKS

In addition to immediate morbidity and mortality, caesarean births are linked to significant long-term health issues. They elevate the risk of future infertility, placental abnormalities, uterine rupture, and stillbirth. The likelihood of conditions such as placenta previa, placenta accreta, and placental abruption also rises in subsequent pregnancies. Specifically, the risk of placenta accreta increases from 3% after the first caesarean to 11% after the second, 40% after the third, and 60% after the fourth caesarean section. Additionally, women with a history of caesarean delivery face a higher risk of complications if they require a hysterectomy later in life.

Concerns about newborn safety have contributed to the rising rates of caesarean sections. While elective caesarean deliveries may reduce the risk of intrapartum asphyxia, they are associated with a higher incidence of respiratory complications at birth, even among term infants. The risk of fetal lacerations during caesarean delivery is about 2%. Additionally, iatrogenic prematurity remains a significant issue, as clinicians sometimes fail to adjust gestational dates based on ultrasound findings when discrepancies arise with menstrual dates. To minimize the risk of neonatal respiratory distress syndrome, elective caesarean sections should ideally be performed at 39 completed weeks or later. Long-term risks associated with caesarean births include potential alterations in immune development, an increased likelihood of allergies, atopy, and asthma, as well as changes in gut microbiota in infants, which may predispose them to obesity and metabolic syndrome later in life.

REFERENCES

1. Committee on Practice Bulletins-Obstetrics. Practice Bulletin No. 183: Postpartum Hemorrhage. Obstet Gynecol. 2017;130(4):e168-86.
2. Clark SL, Belfort MA, Dildy GA, Herbst MA, Meyers JA, Hankins GD. Maternal death in the 21st century: causes, prevention, and relationship to cesarean delivery. Am J Obstet Gynecol. 2008;199(1):36.e1-36.e5.
3. Liu S, Liston RM, Joseph KS, Heaman M, Sauve R, Kramer MS, et al. Maternal mortality and severe morbidity associated with low-risk planned cesarean delivery versus planned vaginal delivery at term. Can Med Assoc J. 2007;176(4):455-60.

CHAPTER 4

Preoperative Preparation

INTRODUCTION

Preoperative assessment and optimization of patient, where times allows, is important. Laboratory investigations, anesthesia assessment, especially in high risk cases, is crucial. Cross matching adequate blood and blood products should be done before a caesarean birth.

INDICATIONS

The most common indications for caesarean sections include fetal distress, failure to progress in labor, repeat caesarean deliveries, and breech presentation. In recent years, maternal requests have also emerged as a significant reason for the procedure.

There are two main absolute indications for a caesarean section, even in cases of known fetal abnormalities: central placenta previa and gross pelvic contraction. In most other situations involving fetal abnormalities, efforts should be made to achieve a vaginal delivery, unless the abnormality can be corrected after birth, and a caesarean section would improve fetal survival.

Indications for caesarean sections are generally categorized into absolute and relative. Relative indications can be further divided into elective (planned) and nonelective (emergent) cases. **Table 1** highlights indications of caesarean section.

PREOPERATIVE MEASURES

Among all measures, the most crucial is to rule out anemia or treat it if time allows. If there has been acute blood loss prior to the operation, it should be replaced; however, a caesarean should not be postponed if the patient is actively bleeding. It is essential to find out the blood group and cross match and save. In case of abnormal antibodies, weekly cross matching should be done.

The stomach should be empty before a caesarean section. Gastric emptying is often delayed during labor, especially in cases where the patient has been in labor for some time and has been taking food or fluids orally, increasing the risk of aspiration of acidic gastric contents during anesthesia. This can lead to chemical aspiration pneumonitis, known as Mendelson syndrome. To minimize this risk, solid foods should be avoided during

TABLE 1: Indications for caesarean section.[1,2]

Maternal indications	*Uterine/anatomic indications*	*Fetal indications*
Prior caesarean delivery	Abnormal placentation such as placenta previa and placenta accreta	Nonreassuring fetal status (e.g., abnormal umbilical cord on Doppler study) or abnormal fetal heart tracing
Maternal request	Placental abruption	Umbilical cord prolapse
Pelvic deformity or cephalopelvic disproportion	Prior classical hysterotomy	Failed operative vaginal delivery
Previous perineal trauma	Prior full-thickness myomectomy	Malpresentation
Prior pelvic or anal/rectal reconstructive surgery	History of uterine incision dehiscence	Macrosomia
Active genital primary herpes simplex	Invasive cervical cancer	Congenital anomaly like conjoint twins
Cardiac or pulmonary disease	Prior trachelectomy	Thrombocytopenia
Cerebral aneurysm or arteriovenous malformation	Obstructive mass in the genital tract	
Pathology requiring concurrent intraabdominal surgery	Permanent cerclage	
Perimortem caesarean		

active labor, and patients should be H2 receptor antagonists or proton pump inhibitors to reduce gastric volume and acidity, as well as anti-emetics prior to the procedure.

Informed written consent should be obtained after clearly explaining the reasons for the caesarean section, along with the associated risks and benefits for both the mother and the fetus. Additionally, the American College of Obstetricians and Gynecologists (ACOG) provides a checklist for planned caesarean deliveries that should be followed for all patients.

ANAESTHESIA

The risk of anesthesia-related deaths during caesarean sections is notably higher in low- and middle-income countries. A meta-analysis found that anesthesia was responsible for 13.8% of maternal deaths following caesarean deliveries. General anesthesia significantly increased the odds of maternal and perinatal deaths compared to neuraxial anesthesia. Complications related to general anesthesia, such as failed intubation, inadequate ventilation and oxygenation, and pulmonary aspiration of gastric contents, were the leading causes of these deaths.[3] Additionally, severe morbidity was more common among women receiving general anesthesia compared to those with neuraxial techniques.

The majority of caesarean sections today are performed under regional anesthesia. Indications for general anesthesia are limited and include acute severe fetal distress, acute maternal hypovolemia, failed regional anesthesia, significant coagulopathy, and maternal refusal of regional anesthesia. General anesthesia should ideally be avoided in patients with severe asthma, a history of malignant hyperthermia, or those with difficult airways.

Local anesthesia can serve as a safe and effective alternative when regional or general anesthesia is unavailable or when trained personnel are not present. The World Health Organization recognizes local anesthesia for caesarean sections in its evidence-based practical manual, recommending its use by trained and experienced practitioners. However, this approach should be avoided in women with eclampsia or severe pre-eclampsia, those who are obese, apprehensive, allergic to lignocaine, or if the surgeon lacks experience.

REFERENCES

1. Barber EL, Lundsberg LS, Belanger K, Pettker CM, Funai EF, Illuzzi JL. Indications Contributing to the Increasing Cesarean Delivery Rate. Obstet Gynecol. 2011;118(1):29-38.
2. Boyle A, Reddy UM, Landy HJ, Huang CC, Driggers RW, Laughon SK. Primary Cesarean Delivery in the United States. Obstet Gynecol. 2013;122(1):33-40.
3. Hawkins JL, Koonin LM, Palmer SK, Gibbs CP. Anesthesia-related Deaths during Obstetric Delivery in the United States, 1979–1990. Anesthesiology. 1997;86(2):277-84.

5

CHAPTER

Technique of Caesarean Section

INTRODUCTION

The technique for caesarean section has evolved over time. From sharp dissection to bluntly opening the abdomen, obstetricians have their own preferences. The Misgav Ladach method is faster and more popular. The technique for closure of uterine incision and layers of the abdomen may also vary.

CLASSICAL CAESAREAN SECTION

The indications for caesarean sections in modern obstetrics are quite limited and include:

- Postmortem caesarean section
- Moribund patient with antepartum hemorrhage
- Inaccessible lower segment due to dense adhesions or myoma in the lower uterine segment
- Occasionally, in cases of transverse lie with neglected shoulder presentation
- Severe kyphosis where the distance between the sternum and pubis is significantly reduced
- Cancer of the cervix

  Figures 1A to C showing various uterine incisions during caesarean section.

TECHNIQUE OF LOWER SEGMENT CAESAREAN SECTION

During the operation, the patient should be positioned supine with a left-lateral tilt of 10–15 degrees. It is essential to check the fetal heart rate before starting the surgery. After cleaning and draping the patient, the surgeon should examine the abdomen to confirm the baby's position. Bladder catheterization before surgery is not mandatory; there is no consensus on its necessity. A case-control study indicated that women who were not catheterized experienced earlier ambulation, less voiding discomfort, and a lower incidence of urinary tract infections (UTIs). However, larger randomized studies are needed to clarify this issue. If a catheter is used, it is not beneficial to keep it in place for >12 hours.

Abdominal Incision (Fig. 2)

The commonly used incisions for caesarean sections include the Pfannenstiel incision, the Joel–Cohen incision, and low vertical incisions.

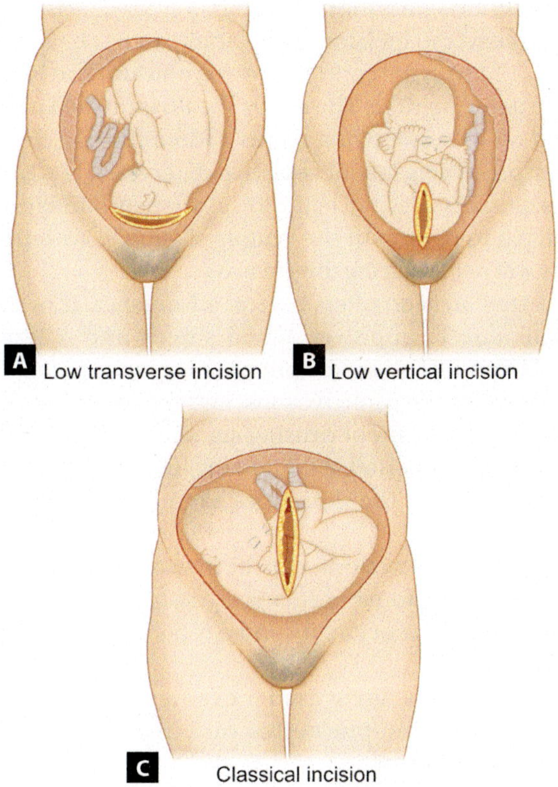

Figs. 1A to C: Uterine incisions during caesarean section.
Source: https://www.mayoclinic.org/-/media/kcms/gbs/patient- consumer/images/2013/11/15/17/38/my00214_-my00642_im03562_pr7_csection_uterthu_jpg.jpg

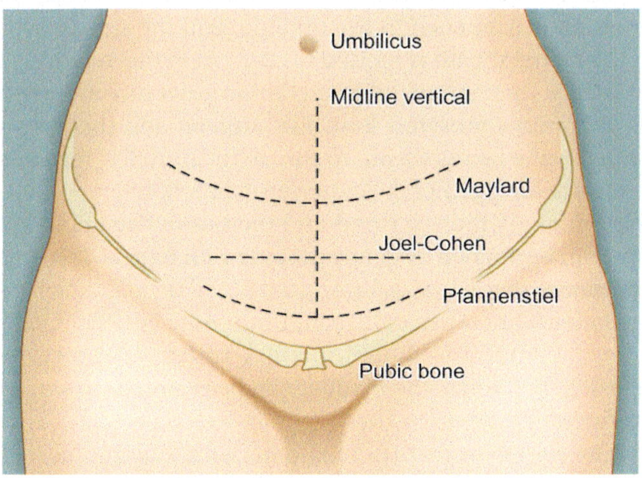

Fig. 2: Various abdominal incisions useful for caesarean section.
Source: Figures taken from https://epos.myesr.org/posterimage/esr/ecr2019/148981/mediagallery/827100?deliveroriginal=1.

The Pfannenstiel incision is the most commonly used incision for caesarean sections. It is a transverse incision made about 2 cm above the symphysis pubis, slightly curved with the concavity facing upward, and its midpoint is at or just below the pubic hairline. The rectus sheath is divided transversely and carefully peeled off the underlying rectus abdominis muscles using blunt-pointed scissors, preserving lateral vessels and nerves. It is advisable to leave the pyramidalis muscles attached to the lower aponeurotic flap and to bluntly dissect them down to the top of the symphysis pubis. With practice, fewer bleeding points will occur during this incision.

The Pfannenstiel incision offers several advantages. It heals better than vertical incisions due to improved blood supply and is less affected by increased intra-abdominal pressure from straining or coughing. Postoperative pain is also reduced for the same reasons, and the fundus of the uterus can be palpated more easily without causing significant discomfort during the immediate postoperative period. Additionally, because the incision follows the natural lines of Langer, the skin edges align better, resulting in a more cosmetic scar.

Repeat Pfannenstiel incisions can be performed without difficulty, and the incidence of incisional hernia is significantly lower with this type of incision. If a hernia does occur, it can be repaired concurrently with the caesarean delivery.

The Maylard incision is rarely used for caesarean sections. It is similar to the Pfannenstiel incision, but in this case, the rectus muscles are cut transversely to enhance access.

Joel–Cohen Incision

The Joel–Cohen incision was introduced by Joel Cohen in 1972. It is a transverse straight abdominal incision made 2–3 cm above the Pfannenstiel incision site. The incision is deepened in the midline, and the subcutaneous tissue along with the rectus sheath is incised for 2–3 cm in this relatively avascular area. The fascia is then stretched in a craniocaudal direction between the two rectus abdominis muscles. Both the surgeon and the assistant place two fingers below the rectus sheath to stretch the muscles, rectus fascia, and subcutaneous tissues together in a transverse direction.

The peritoneum is then grasped and incised in the upper third of the incision, or it can be opened by gently probing with fingers. It is crucial not to incise the peritoneum too low, as during labor or late pregnancy, the bladder may be positioned higher than anticipated and could be accidentally opened. If this occurs, the procedure should continue with the delivery of the baby, and after closing the uterus, the bladder can be repaired in two layers using 3-0 vicryl sutures.

A Cochrane review from 2013 included two trials comparing the Joel–Cohen incision to the Pfannenstiel incision, showing that the Joel–Cohen incision resulted in less postoperative fever, reduced pain and analgesic needs, less blood loss, and shorter surgery and hospital stays.[1]

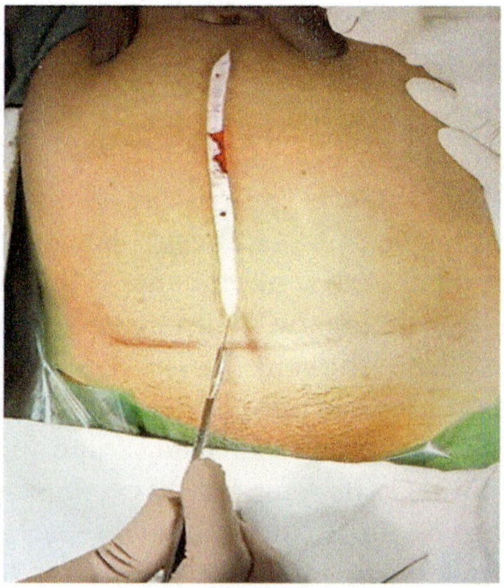

Fig. 3: Vertical abdominal incision.

Lower Vertical Incision

The low vertical incision is rarely used today and can be either midline or paramedian. It provides quicker access to the lower uterine segment, better exposure, and less blood loss. However, vertical skin incisions **(Fig. 3)** are associated with a higher risk of incisional hernias compared to transverse incisions. Currently, the only valid indications for using a vertical incision are the concurrent removal of a large ovarian cyst or in rare cases where a classical caesarean section is required.

Correcting Dextrorotation

Dextrorotation of the uterus should be addressed, as it positions the highly vascular left lateral border of the uterus in the incision line. If large veins are visible on the surface of the uterus, it is advisable to suspect this rotation and confirm it by inserting a hand to feel for the round ligaments and make the necessary corrections. While it may not always be possible to perfectly centralize the uterus, being aware of this anatomical variation allows the incision to be initiated further to the right, bringing it closer to the uterine midline.

IDENTIFICATION OF THE LOWER SEGMENT

Identifying the upper margin of the lower segment of the uterus is straightforward. This margin is where the serous coat of the anterior wall becomes less tightly attached to the underlying muscle, allowing it to be moved more easily. During labor, this limit is significantly elevated. However, in the absence of contractions, in cases of prematurity, transverse lie, or placenta previa, the lower segment can be much shorter, increasing the risk of inadvertently incising too high, possibly even into the upper segment of the uterus.

BLADDER FLAP DEVELOPMENT

The upper edge of the bladder typically lies about 5 cm below the demarcation line of the lower segment, which is usually visible as a distinct groove. To begin, the peritoneum of the uterovesical fold is grasped in the midline with forceps and incised with scissors. The scissors should be inserted beneath the peritoneum on both sides to open the areolar space and ensure there's no risk of injuring the bladder. The peritoneum is then cut transversely in a curved manner, almost reaching the round ligaments laterally, while being careful not to damage the uterine veins.

Beneath this incision, a layer of thin connective tissue will be encountered, which should also be grasped and incised. Some venous bleeding may occur at this stage, but it can be temporarily overlooked. The lower flap of the peritoneum, along with the bladder, is then reflected down to expose a sufficient area of the lower segment for the incision.

In cases of repeat caesarean sections, the bladder may adhere to the lower uterine segment, making sharp dissection preferable to blunt dissection. In such instances, adhesions should be stretched and incised with scissors to facilitate cleavage.

The necessity of developing a bladder flap before making the uterine incision has been explored in several randomized trials. One study indicated that omitting the bladder flap could reduce both operating time and blood loss, while a subsequent larger trial found no significant differences in total operating time or complications between groups.[2]

Currently, there is insufficient evidence to determine whether creating a bladder flap offers any clear advantages **(Fig. 4)**.

Uterine Incision

This is the most commonly performed incision. The Doyen retractor is re-applied after incising the ureterovesical peritoneum to retract the

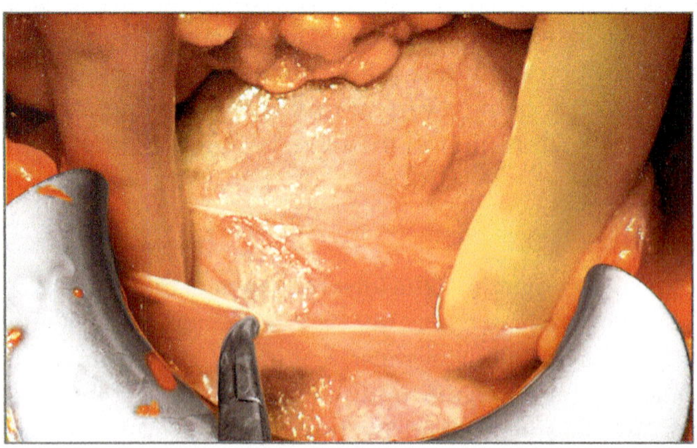

Fig. 4: Bladder flap development.

bladder with it. A stab incision is made in the midline about 2 cm wide. The incision is then increased manually by inserting the index fingers of both hands. Alternatively, two fingers of the left hand can be inserted through the incision between the membranes and the lower segment. These fingers raise the uterine wall and protect the underlying fetus and the incision is then extended laterally in each direction with curved scissors, concavity directed upwards **(Fig. 2)**. It is best to try to leave the membranes intact at this stage in order to avoid the risk of cutting the baby and to maintain the liquor until the uterine incision **(Fig. 5)** is completed.

Occasionally, some large veins may be seen coursing over the lower uterine segment. If possible, they should be avoided in making the incision. If it is not possible to avoid, the large vessels can be under-run and tied below and above the incision line. By adopting the above precautions, one should seldom encounter severe hemorrhage from the lateral angles or an incision that has gone too far outward.

A great proportion of the muscle fibers low down in the lower segment are arranged in a circular fashion so that a transverse scar is more suitable anatomically. It is also easier to control the extent of a transverse incision, whereas a vertical one may accidentally be extended too far downwards behind the bladder and it is often difficult to make a large enough opening without encroaching on the upper uterine segment, thereby defeating the whole purpose of the lower segment operation. Specific dangers are injury to vessels at lateral margins of the uterus, hemorrhage, and hematoma at angles.

The upper edge of the bladder typically lies about 5 cm below the demarcation line of the lower segment, which is usually visible as a distinct groove. To begin, the peritoneum of the uterovesical fold is grasped in the midline with forceps and incised with scissors. The scissors should be inserted beneath the peritoneum on both sides to open the areolar space

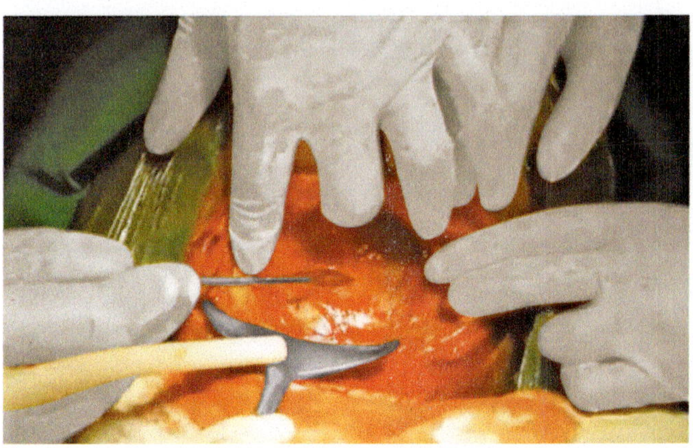

Fig. 5: Uterine incision.

and ensure there's no risk of injuring the bladder. The peritoneum is then cut transversely in a curved manner, almost reaching the round ligaments laterally, while being careful not to damage the uterine veins. Beneath this incision, a layer of thin connective tissue will be encountered, which should also be grasped and incised. Some venous bleeding may occur at this stage, but it can be temporarily overlooked. The lower flap of the peritoneum, along with the bladder, is then reflected down to expose a sufficient area of the lower segment for the incision.

In cases of repeat caesarean sections, the bladder may adhere to the lower uterine segment, making sharp dissection preferable to blunt dissection. In such instances, adhesions should be stretched and incised with scissors to facilitate cleavage.

The necessity of developing a bladder flap before making the uterine incision has been explored in several randomized trials. One study indicated that omitting the bladder flap could reduce both operating time and blood loss, while a subsequent larger trial found no significant differences in total operating time or complications between groups. Currently, there is insufficient evidence to determine whether creating a bladder flap offers any clear advantages.

DELIVERY OF HEAD

Once the uterus is opened, the Doyen retractor is removed to create space for the surgeon's hand. The hand should be carefully guided beneath the fetal head **(Fig. 6)** to encourage maximum flexion, allowing smaller diameters to pass through the incision. If the vertex is deeply engaged, having a scrubbed assistant with a hand in the vagina to gently push the head upward can facilitate delivery. This approach is preferable to forcibly dislodging the head from above, which risks extending the incision into surrounding vessels or the vaginal area, potentially leading to serious complications.

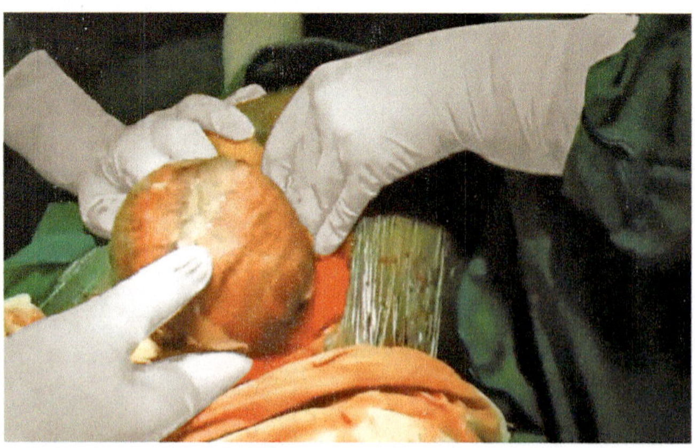

Fig. 6: Delivery of fetal head.

In situations where a hand cannot be placed below the fetal head, one blade of forceps can be inserted as a Vectis to assist in delivery. For a high, free-floating head, using Wrigley forceps may provide a more straightforward method than trying to grasp the head manually.

Once the head is delivered, the anesthetist should start an intravenous infusion of 10 units of oxytocin in 500 mL of Ringer's lactate. Alternatively, 5–10 units of oxytocin can be given intramuscularly. This step is crucial, as it significantly reduces blood loss.

When delivering the shoulders, it's best to elevate the head to allow the posterior shoulder to emerge first. There's no need to rush this process; rough handling may lead to tearing of the lower segment. The rest of the baby's body should be delivered slowly and with care.

As soon as the head is delivered, the anesthetist should initiate an intravenous infusion of 10 units of oxytocin in 500 mL of Ringer's lactate, or administer 5–10 units intramuscularly. This crucial step significantly reduces blood loss.

For delivering the shoulders, it's advisable to raise the head to allow the posterior shoulder to emerge first. There's no need to rush; gentle handling is essential to prevent tearing of the lower segment. The rest of the baby's body should then be delivered slowly and carefully.

THIRD STAGES

If the preceding steps **(Fig. 7)** have been executed properly, there should be minimal bleeding, allowing for a brief wait of one to two minutes for the

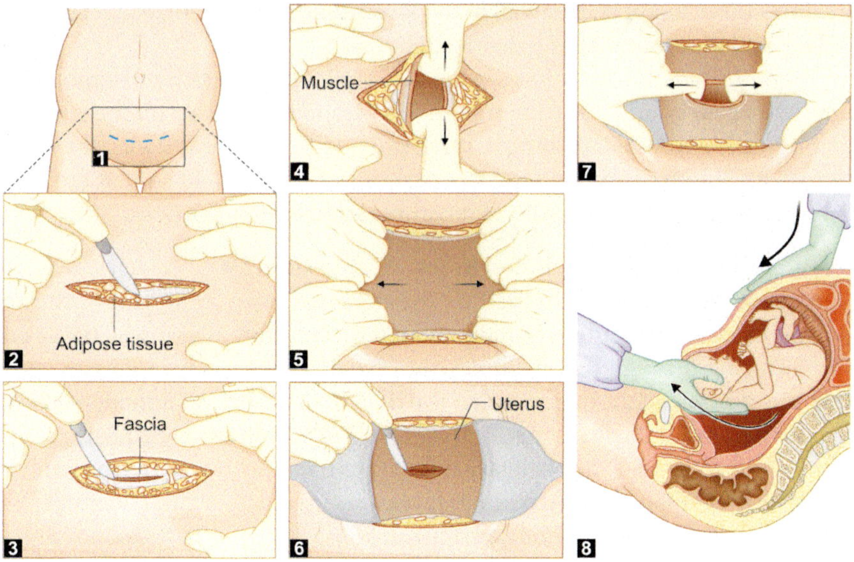

Fig. 7: Steps of caesarean section.
Source: Figure taken from https://encrypted-tbn2.gstatic.com/images?q=tbn:ANd9GcRwfOV7_ylby0wh-J-IQEkJMDFubkf3NilFGmFDSgslg_qzMG7B.

placenta to separate spontaneously. While some obstetricians routinely perform manual removal of the placenta, this is generally unnecessary and can lead to increased bleeding compared to allowing for natural separation.

A recent Cochrane review has indicated that manual removal is associated with a higher incidence of endometritis, greater maternal blood loss (over 1,000 mL), a more significant drop in hematocrit after delivery, and prolonged hospital stays. However, the evidence regarding differences in fetomaternal hemorrhage between the two methods remains inconclusive.

Spontaneous delivery of the placenta, supported by gentle controlled cord traction, should be encouraged. Care should be taken to avoid pulling on the cord before the placenta has separated, as this could risk uterine inversion through the lower segment incision, potentially leading to hypotension.

CLOSURE OF UTERINE INCISION

After delivering the placenta, the Doyen retractor is repositioned to allow for inspection of the uterine incision. Any bleeding edges should be held with Green-Armytage hemostatic forceps; ideally, four forceps are placed—one at each angle of the incision and one at both the upper and lower margins, though a minimum of two at the angles is required. Some surgeons prefer using Allis forceps due to their lighter weight and less intrusive nature.

It's crucial to accurately identify the lower edge of the uterine incision, which can sometimes retract behind the bladder or be obscured by blood in the pelvis. A common and hazardous mistake is suturing the upper edge of the incision to the posterior wall of the lower uterine segment, especially if it bulges into the wound after placenta delivery.

A continuous suture is initiated at one angle of the incision. Hemostasis relies more on good approximation of the wound edges than on the specific technique used. While locking sutures provide better hemostasis, they can impair healing by strangulating the tissues. An absorbable suture, such as Vicryl 1-0 on an eyeless needle, is recommended for this purpose.

Should the decidua be included in the uterine suture?

The question of whether to include the decidual layer in uterine suturing during caesarean sections remains debated. Traditionally, it was believed that suturing through the decidua could create pathways for infection and that the sutures might loosen when the decidua is shed, potentially leading to poor healing of the uterine scar. However, a recent study using postpartum ultrasound six weeks after delivery found that full-thickness suturing, which includes the endometrial (decidual) layer, was associated with fewer defects at the incision site compared to split-thickness suturing that excluded the endometrial layer. Ongoing randomized trials aim to provide clearer guidance on this issue and determine the best practice for suturing techniques in caesarean deliveries.

EXTRA-ABDOMINAL VERSUS INTRA-ABDOMINAL REPAIR OF THE UTERINE INCISION

There is currently no definitive evidence to favor one uterine repair technique over another in caesarean sections. A review of recent randomized controlled trials (RCTs) reveals mixed findings: one RCT indicated that intra-abdominal repair resulted in lower rates of nausea and vomiting and quicker recovery of bowel function compared to exteriorizing the uterus for repair.[3] Conversely, another RCT noted reduced mean blood loss with extra-abdominal repair but found no significant differences in other outcomes.[4]

In cases of excessive bleeding, exteriorizing the uterus may provide better visibility for identifying and repairing bleeding edges. However, further studies with larger participant groups are needed to ascertain any substantial differences in operative and postoperative morbidity between these two techniques.

Single- versus Two-layer Suturing for Uterine Closure

The traditional approach to suturing the uterine incision after a caesarean section involves two layers **(Fig. 8)**: The first layer approximates the bulk of the uterine muscle, while the second uses inverting or Lembert sutures

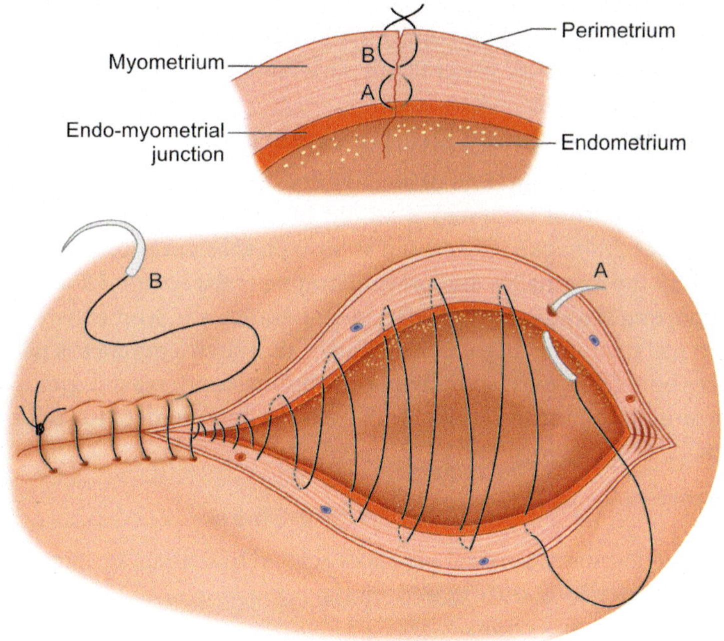

Fig. 8: Double layer uterine closure.
Source: Figure taken from https://encrypted-tbn0.gstatic.com/images?q=tbn:ANd9GcQo11_AlwdKNPa28yxiwClhNUBJyqRTlu1TEA&s.

to bury the first layer **(Fig. 4)**. However, some have proposed single-layer closure to potentially reduce operating time, minimize tissue disruption, and decrease the amount of foreign material introduced into the wound, which could enhance healing and reduce postoperative complications.

A recent meta-analysis comparing uterine closure techniques found that double-layer unlocked sutures are preferable to single-layer locked sutures.[5] This preference is based on findings related to residual myometrial thickness and the incidence of dysmenorrhea. The analysis also indicated that excluding the decidua during suturing is associated with a higher prevalence of uterine niches—defects in the caesarean scar linked to poorer scar integrity. These niches may increase the risk of complications such as postmenstrual spotting, uterine dehiscence, and caesarean scar pregnancy.

Closure versus Nonclosure of the Peritoneum

The 2014 Cochrane review on the closure versus nonclosure of the peritoneum found that nonclosure can lead to reduced operative time and shorter postoperative stays.[5] However, the evidence regarding adhesion formation and other outcomes was inconsistent. A RCT comparing the two methods indicated that closing both peritoneal layers was associated with higher postoperative pain scores, as well as increased pulse rates and blood pressure in that group. As a result, the current clinical recommendation favors nonclosure of both visceral and parietal peritoneum.[6]

Cervical Dilatation during Elective Caesarean

Cervical dilatation at the time of elective caesarean section in women with undilated cervix (not in labor) is an old practice that was undertaken to ensure proper drainage of lochia. It was thought that a portion of the chorion may overlap the internal os and prevent drainage. Except for a few anecdotal cases reporting the absence of lochia postoperatively in women who did not have cervical dilatation, there is no evidence that such a practice is necessary or of any benefit. It may actually contribute to an increased incidence of postpartum endometritis, although there is no definite data to support this concern.

INSPECTION AND CLOSURE OF ABDOMEN

The passage discusses surgical practices related to managing complications and closing incisions during abdominal procedures, particularly in the context of caesarean sections.

- *Hematoma management:* Blood accumulation (hematoma) can occur, especially at the incision corners, often due to vein puncture. Mattress sutures can help control this.

- *Field cleaning:* It is crucial to clear blood from the surgical field, including areas like the paracolic gutters and behind the uterus. Inspection of the tubes and ovaries for incidental findings is also performed.
- *Peritoneal irrigation:* Although irrigation of the peritoneal cavity may be done before closing the abdomen, studies show it doesn't significantly impact postoperative outcomes.
- *Rectus muscle closure:* There's no consensus on reapproximating the rectus muscles, as suturing may cause postoperative pain. Most surgeons opt not to suture them.
- *Layered closure:* The abdominal wall is closed in layers: Rectus sheath, subcutaneous fat, and skin. Proper closure of the rectus sheath is vital for abdominal wall strength.

The closure of the subcutaneous fat layer during a caesarean section has been shown to help minimize the risk of hematomas and seromas, particularly when the fat layer exceeds 2 cm.[7] Skin closure can be performed using various techniques, including subcuticular stitches (absorbable or nonabsorbable), interrupted sutures (usually nonabsorbable), or skin staples. Despite the variety of methods, there is no strong evidence indicating that one technique is superior to others. For patients prone to keloids, a subcuticular suture with nonabsorbable materials like nylon or Prolene, with delayed removal of sutures (up to 4 weeks), may be beneficial. Unsightly scars should be excised, while well-healed scars can be left intact. Drains may be utilized in specific cases, such as poor hemostasis, obesity, or previous surgeries. Before concluding the procedure, the surgeon should ensure that the uterus is well contracted, clean the vagina, and remove any blood clots. If an indwelling catheter is in place, checking the urine for blood can help confirm that the bladder is intact, although slight hematuria may occur from bladder retraction during surgery.

An occlusive dressing is typically applied for the first 48 hours postsurgery. Since epithelialization generally occurs within 24–48 hours, the dressing can usually be removed after this period. The wound should then be inspected for signs of infection, hematoma, or dehiscence. Based on the wound's condition and the patient's comfort, a nonocclusive dressing may be applied, or the wound may be left open. Some surgeons choose not to change the dressing if there are no indications of infection, allowing it to remain for up to 7 days before removal and subsequent stitch removal if necessary.

MODIFIED TECHNIQUE FOR LOWER SEGMENT CAESAREAN SECTION: THE MISGAV LADACH METHOD

The Misgav Ladach method, introduced by Dr Michael Stark and colleagues at Misgav Ladach Hospital in Jerusalem, focuses on minimizing tissue trauma through reduced dissection.[1] Key steps in this technique include:

Joel Cohen skin incision: A specific type of incision designed for minimal trauma.

↓

Digital opening of the parietal peritoneum: This is done at the upper intermuscular space, stretching it in a cranial-caudal direction.

↓

Bladder displacement: The ureterovesical fold is opened, and the bladder is pushed down using blunt dissection.

↓

Lower uterine segment incision: A small transverse incision is made, allowing for two fingers to fit, and this incision is manually stretched.

↓

Single-layer uterine closure: The uterus is closed with a single layer, although this approach is not recommended as standard practice.

↓

Unsutured peritoneum: Both parietal and visceral peritoneum are left unsutured. Two-layer abdominal closure: The abdominal wall is closed in two layers, involving the rectus sheath and skin.

Several prospective studies indicate that caesarean sections performed using the Misgav Ladach technique result in reduced operative time, less blood loss, lower postoperative analgesia needs, decreased febrile morbidity, and shorter hospital stays compared to the conventional Pfannenstiel method. However, the single-layer uterine closure remains a point of contention and is not advised for routine use.

REFERENCES

1. Vardhan S, Behera R, Kathpalia S, Bhattacharya T. Modified Technique of LSCS: The Misgav Ladach Method. Med J Armed Forces India. 2005;61(3):271-2.
2. Smith J, Jones D, Thompson P, Green M. Bladder flap omission in hysterectomy: A randomized controlled trial of its effect on operative time and blood loss. J Surg Res. 2017;125(4):415-21.
3. Abdellah MS, Abbas AM, Ali MK, Mahmoud A, Abdullah SA. Uterine exteriorization versus intraperitoneal repair: effect on intraoperative nausea and vomiting during repeat cesarean delivery - A randomized clinical trial. Facts Views Vis Ob Gyn. 2018;10(3):131-7.

4. Zaphiratos V, George RB, Boyd JC, Habib AS. Uterine exteriorization compared with in situ repair for cesarean delivery: a systematic review and meta-analysis. Obstet Anesth Dig. 2016;36(3):137-8.
5. Qayum K, Kar I, Sofi J, Panneerselvam H. Single- versus double-layer uterine closure after cesarean section delivery: a systematic review and meta-analysis. Cureus. 2021;13(9):e18405.
6. Bamigboye AA, Hofmeyr GJ. Closure versus non-closure of the peritoneum at caesarean section. Cochrane Database Syst Rev. 2003:(4):CD000163.
7. National Institute for Health and Care Excellence. (2021). Caesarean birth [NICE Guideline No. 192]. [online] Available from https://www.nice.org.uk/guidance/ng192 [Last accessed December, 2024].

CHAPTER 6

Postoperative Care

INTRODUCTION

Postoperative care for patients undergoing caesarean sections includes fluid management, venous thromboembolism risk assessment and prevention and optimizing the patient by enhanced recovery after surgery pathway.

POSTOPERATIVE PAIN

Adequate pain relief postcaesarean section (CS) can be achieved through methods such as topping up epidural analgesia, using patient-controlled analgesia, or administering injectable nonsteroidal anti-inflammatory drugs (NSAIDs) or narcotic analgesics as needed.[1] Monitoring should include vital signs, uterine contractions, and vaginal bleeding every half hour for the first 2 hours, then hourly until the patient stabilizes. If epidural opioids are used, monitoring should continue for at least 2 hours after the analgesia is stopped.

Urinary catheters can be removed once the patient is mobile following regional anesthesia, but not sooner than 12 hours after the last top-up. Clear fluids may be introduced as early as 2 hours postsurgery, and if tolerated, solid food can be gradually added. A recent Cochrane review supports early intake of oral fluids and food, noting that it aids in the return of bowel activity and that withholding oral intake post-uncomplicated CS is unnecessary.

Routine complete blood count (CBC) testing the day after surgery was once standard, but it may not be needed for all women. Testing is advisable for those who experience significant blood loss (≥1,000 mL) or who are already anemic. Blood transfusions should only be considered if hemoglobin levels fall below 7 g/dL, as smaller blood losses can often be managed with a good diet along with iron and folic acid supplementation.

THROMBOPROPHYLAXIS

In developed countries, where maternal mortality from hemorrhage and infection has been significantly reduced, venous thromboembolism (VTE)—which includes deep vein thrombosis (DVT) and pulmonary embolism—has become a major cause of maternal death. The risk of VTE following a CS is approximately twice that of vaginal delivery (VD) and is even higher after emergency CSs.

The risk of VTE is four times higher after a CS compared to a VD. This increased risk appears to be independent of other VTE risk factors and is higher after an emergency CS than an elective CS. On average, 3 out of every 1,000 women will develop VTE following a CS.[2] This highlights the increased risk associated with surgical delivery methods, particularly in emergency situations.

International guidelines regarding pharmacological thromboprophylaxis [low-molecular-weight heparin (LMWH)] after caesarean births vary significantly. A study comparing eligibility for postcaesarean LMWH based on the guidelines from the Royal College of Obstetricians and Gynaecologists (RCOG), the American College of Chest Physicians (Chest), and the American College of Obstetricians and Gynecologists (ACOG) found that 85%, 34.8%, and 1.0% of women, respectively, would qualify for treatment.[3] The most recent RCOG guidelines recommend considering LMWH for all women following a CS for 10 days to reduce the incidence of VTE.

However, while LMWH may reduce VTE risks, it also increases the likelihood of hemorrhage and wound complications. Given the low occurrence of clinical events and the potential for harm, universal pharmacological thromboprophylaxis is not justified for all women undergoing CSs. Encouraging early ambulation can help minimize thromboembolism risks postpartum. Additionally, the use of pneumatic compression stockings is an effective method for thromboprophylaxis and can reduce the risk of fatal VTE. According to ACOG recommendations, the following approaches should be taken for thromboprophylaxis after caesarean births:[3]

- Perioperative mechanical thromboprophylaxis is recommended for all women.
- Pharmacological prophylaxis (LMWH or unfractionated heparin) is advised for those with:
    - High-risk thrombophilias
    - Previous VTE events
    - Family history of VTE and thrombophilia
    - Multiple risk factors, including obesity or prolonged immobility

The LMWH should ideally be started 6–12 hours after the caesarean. Both oral anticoagulants and heparin are considered safe for breastfeeding, which can begin as soon as the operating room. If recovery is uneventful, patients may be safely discharged by the third postoperative day, promoting a quicker return to their normal environment, enhancing psychological well-being, and reducing the risk of nosocomial infections.

PROPHYLACTIC ANTIBIOTICS

Antibiotics are recommended for both elective and nonelective CSs, as they have been shown to significantly reduce the incidence of endometritis, wound infections, and serious infections by 60–70%. A recent Cochrane review (2018) suggests that vaginal preparation with povidone-iodine or chlorhexidine solution—compared to saline or no cleansing—likely reduces the risk of postcaesarean endometritis.[4] This benefit appears to be particularly pronounced for women who are in labor or have ruptured membranes.

Many antibiotic regimens have been reported to be effective for prophylaxis during CSs. A common approach involves administering a single dose of both ampicillin and a first-generation cephalosporin, such as cefazolin. This combination has been shown to effectively reduce the risk of postoperative infections, including endometritis and wound infections. Other regimens may also be used depending on specific patient factors and local guidelines. Overall, the goal is to provide adequate coverage to prevent infections in the postoperative period. Effective and there does not seem to be any added benefit in routinely using more broad-spectrum antibiotics or multiple-dose regimens for prophylaxis. However, there is also a suggestion that adding azithromycin to the cephalosporin may reduce the risk of postpartum endometritis. The optimum timing for administration of antibiotics, whether it should be given before the skin incision as is the practice for other surgical procedures, or immediately after the cord is clamped, has been debated for some time. Although there are concerns of a negative effect on infant microbiota, current evidence is in favor of preincision antibiotics, with a lower rate of maternal morbidity and no short-term disadvantage to the neonate. Amoxicillin clavulanate, however, is not recommended if the antibiotic is administered before cord clamping.

REFERENCES

1. National Institute for Health and Care Excellence. (2021). Caesarean birth [NICE Guideline No. 192]. [online] Available from https://www.nice.org.uk/guidance/ng192 [Last accessed December, 2024].
2. Blondon M, Casini A, Hoppe KK, Boehlen F, Righini M, Smith NL. Risks of venous thromboembolism after cesarean sections: a meta-analysis. Chest. 2016;150(3):572-96.
3. Pacheco LD, Saade G, Metz TD. Society for Maternal-Fetal Medicine Consult Series #51: Thromboembolism prophylaxis for cesarean delivery. Am J Obstet Gynecol. 2020;223(2):B11-7.
4. Haas DM, Morgan S, Contreras K, Kimball S. Vaginal preparation with antiseptic solution before cesarean section for preventing postoperative infections. Cochrane Database Syst Rev. 2020;4(4):CD007892.

7

CHAPTER

Complications Associated with Caesarean Sections

INTRODUCTION

It can be categorized into anesthetic, surgical, and those related to preexisting medical or obstetric conditions. These complications may arise either intraoperatively or postoperatively. Some common complications include:

Anesthetic complications:[1]

- *Hypotension:* Often due to regional anesthesia (e.g., epidural or spinal)
- *Allergic reactions:* Rare but possible reactions to anesthetic agents
- *Respiratory issues:* Complications related to general anesthesia

Surgical complications:

- *Infection:* Including endometritis and wound infections
- *Hemorrhage:* Significant blood loss during or after the procedure injury to adjacent organs: Such as the bladder or intestines. Thromboembolic events: Including deep vein thrombosis (DVT) or pulmonary embolism (PE).

Complications related to preexisting conditions:

- *Exacerbation of chronic conditions:* Such as hypertension or diabetes
- *Obstetric complications:* Such as uterine rupture or retained placenta

Monitoring for these complications is essential to ensure timely intervention and improve maternal outcomes.

INTRAOPERATIVE COMPLICATIONS

The overall intraoperative complication rate for caesarean sections is reported to be between 12%, with a significantly higher rate observed in emergency procedures compared to elective ones.[2] The most common intraoperative complications include:

- *Uterocervical lacerations:* These are more likely to occur when the presenting part is deeply engaged in the pelvis, during difficult deliveries, or with larger babies.
- *Hemorrhage:* Blood loss >1,000 mL is more frequently associated with indications such as placenta previa or placental abruption.

Less common complications include injuries to the urinary or gastrointestinal tracts, which may not always be immediately recognized. The prognosis and associated morbidity are significantly better if such injuries are identified and addressed during the same surgical procedure.

Surgeons should exercise heightened caution in cases with increased risk of injury, such as those with a history of previous caesarean sections, pelvic surgery, or multiple abdominal surgeries. If there is any suspicion of injury, it is advisable to take the time to confirm and appropriately manage it, as this can greatly improve outcomes for the patient.

HEMORRHAGE

The average blood loss during a caesarean section is approximately 1,000 mL, which is more than twice that of vaginal delivery. To minimize blood loss, several strategies can be employed:

- *Avoid manual removal of the placenta:* This can help prevent trauma and excessive bleeding.
- *Use of oxytocics:* Administering oxytocin after the delivery of the baby promotes uterine contraction, reducing the risk of hemorrhage.
- *Good surgical technique:* Ensuring proper technique, particularly in securing the angles of the incision and achieving hemostasis, is crucial.
- *Rapid closure of the uterine incision:* Quick and efficient closure of the incision can also help reduce blood loss.

By implementing these practices, the risk of significant hemorrhage during and after the procedure can be effectively minimized. Hemorrhage **(Fig. 1)** after caesarean section can be classified as primary or secondary.

Primary Hemorrhage[3]

This type occurs immediately or shortly after delivery and may result from:

- *Placental bed:* Bleeding can occur from the site where the placenta was attached.

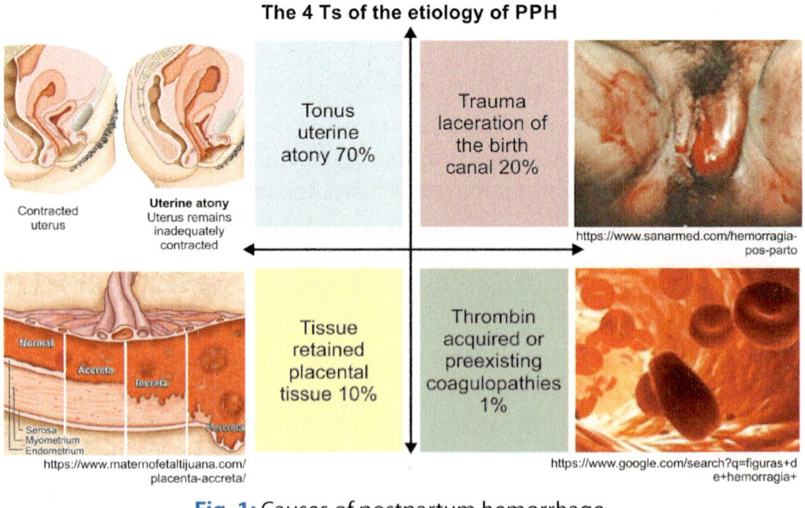

Fig. 1: Causes of postpartum hemorrhage.

Source: Figure taken from https://html.scirp.org/file/8-1442075x21.png?20230830091656801.

- *Tear or extension of the uterine incision:* This may happen during surgery or due to complications postdelivery.

Several factors increase the risk of primary hemorrhage, including:
- General anesthesia
- Placenta previa
- Antepartum hemorrhage
- Macrosomia (large baby)
- Amnionitis (infection of the amniotic fluid)
- Preeclampsia
- Prolonged labor and
- Second-stage arrest

Management

- *Surgical repair:* If a hemorrhage is due to lacerations or extension of the uterine incision, surgical intervention is necessary to repair the damage.
- *Uterine atony:* This is primarily managed with oxytocics to promote uterine contractions. If bleeding persists, additional measures may be required. Effective monitoring and timely intervention are essential to manage and mitigate the risks associated with hemorrhage following caesarean delivery.

URINARY TRACT INFECTIONS

Bladder injury is the most common urinary tract injury associated with caesarean sections, occurring in approximately 0.1–0.3% of cases. The risk of bladder injury is significantly higher in repeat caesarean sections, increasing fourfold compared to primary caesarean deliveries, largely due to the presence of adhesions from previous surgeries. Other pelvic surgeries can also elevate this risk for the same reason.

Bladder Injury

Adhesions: These often form between the bladder and the lower uterine segment, and nearly half of bladder injuries occur during the process of reflecting the bladder down.[4]

Other risk factors:
- Emergency caesarean section
- Prolonged labor before caesarean
- Attempted vaginal birth after caesarean (VBAC)
- Concurrent uterine rupture

Symptoms and Diagnosis

- *Hematuria:* Some degree of hematuria may be observed in the first 24 hours post-surgery, which can raise suspicion for a bladder injury.

However, this is often due to excessive pressure from the Doyen retractor or rough manipulation during the procedure.

- *Diagnosis:* If there is uncertainty about bladder integrity, diagnostic tests such as intravenous injection of indigo carmine or retrograde instillation of methylene blue can confirm an injury.

Management

- *Bladder repair:* If an injury is confirmed, repair is typically performed in two layers using polyglactin 3-0 sutures. A catheter is placed for continuous drainage for 5–7 days.
- *Ureteric injury:* Although rare, ureteric injuries may occur, often during the repair of lateral extensions of the uterine incision. If a ureter is inadvertently tied, it should be freed, and ureteric catheterization is performed. In cases of significant injury where the ureter is cut or crushed, a ureteric anastomosis may be necessary.

Overall, awareness and prompt recognition of these injuries during and after caesarean sections are crucial for effective management and patient outcomes.

The most common infections following caesarean are endometritis, septic pelvic thrombophlebitis, upper respiratory infection, urinary tract infection (UTI), wound infection, and occasionally pelvic abscess. The incidence of endometritis is 10–20 times higher for caesarean section than for vaginal delivery. Infection is usually polymicrobial and pathogens include peptococci, peptostreptococci, group 2 hemolytic streptococci, *E. coli,* and the *Bacteroides* group of organisms. Management is conservative with broad-spectrum antibiotics such as cephalosporins or clindamycin and gentamicin. The use of prophylactic antibiotics reduces the incidence of endometritis by 66–75% and other infective morbidity.

The incidence of wound infection following caesarean is 1–4.5%. Patient may complain of pain at the incision site, there may be local redness and discharge from the wound, and with more serious infection, the stitch line may give way partially or completely. The most common organisms involved are *Staphylococcus aureus*, anaerobes, and gram-negative organisms such as *Streptococcus faecalis*. Wound swab should be sent for culture and sensitivity.

The UTI has shown a downward trend in caesarean deliveries, probably due to better preventive measures. It complicates 1.8–3.3% of women after caesarean birth. The most important etiological factor is the preoperative catheterization. This can be safely avoided at least in women undergoing an elective caesarean section by making them void urine immediately before surgery, without compromising on the safety of the procedure. When catheterization is required, it can be removed immediately after the caesarean, or may be kept no longer than 12 hours. Any fevers call for full investigation, and in every case, a high vaginal or cervical swab together with a midstream specimen of urine should be taken for culture before starting antibiotics.

RESPIRATORY COMPLAINTS

Respiratory complications occur more frequently after abdominal delivery, contributing to about 10% of cases of puerperal pyrexia. These complications are particularly common in:

- Obese patients
- Smokers
- Individuals with preexisting upper respiratory infections
- Patients who receive general anesthesia, as opposed to regional anesthesia

Symptoms

Patients may exhibit:

- Purulent sputum
- Localized chest signs
- Signs of bronchopneumonia

Diagnosis

A chest X-ray may be necessary to confirm the diagnosis of respiratory complications.

Treatment

Management typically includes:

- *Physiotherapy:* To facilitate lung expansion and help clear secretions
- *Antibiotics:* To treat any underlying infection
- Timely recognition and appropriate management of these complications are essential for improving patient outcomes.

PARALYTIC ILEUS

Paralytic ileus, while infrequent after caesarean sections, presents with specific features such as:[5]

- Painless uniform abdominal distension
- Vomiting
- Non-passage of flatus
- Absent bowel sounds
- Electrolyte imbalance

Diagnosis

Differentiating paralytic ileus from intestinal obstruction can be challenging in postoperative patients. A plain abdominal X-ray can assist in diagnosis **(Fig. 2)**:

- *Paralytic ileus* shows gas in both the small and large intestines.
- *Small bowel obstruction* typically shows no gas in the large bowel.

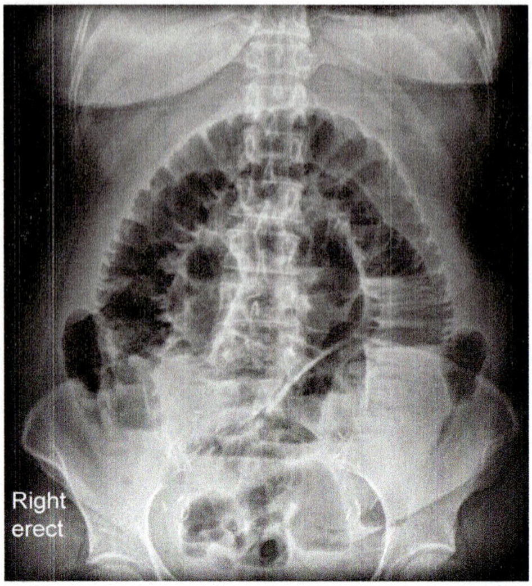

Fig. 2: Diffuse gaseous distension of the small and large bowel loops, accompanied by air-fluid levels on an upright image, is consistent with paralytic ileus, likely related to recent surgery.
Source: Figure taken from https://prod-images-static.radiopaedia.org/images/64210913/82e77c82e17720365416be6896ab0bdb074801c54d2ac5277c97f87c489510fd_big_gallery.jpeg.

Management

Management strategies include:
- *Nil by mouth (NPO):* Keeping the patient without oral intake
- *Gastric decompression:* Using continuous nasogastric drainage

Intravenous Fluids: To maintain hydration and correct any electrolyte imbalances.

Bowel activity usually recovers within 2–3 days, although some cases may require a longer recovery period. Monitoring and supportive care are essential for optimal recovery.

HEMATOMA

The incidence of hematoma after caesarean section is reported to be between 2.4 and 5.6%.

Types of Hematoma

- *Retrovesical hematoma:* This is fairly common following lower segment operations. While it often resolves without significant issues, it can contribute to unexplained postoperative fevers.
- *Hematoma in the abdominal incision:* This may lead to complications such as dehiscence or infection.

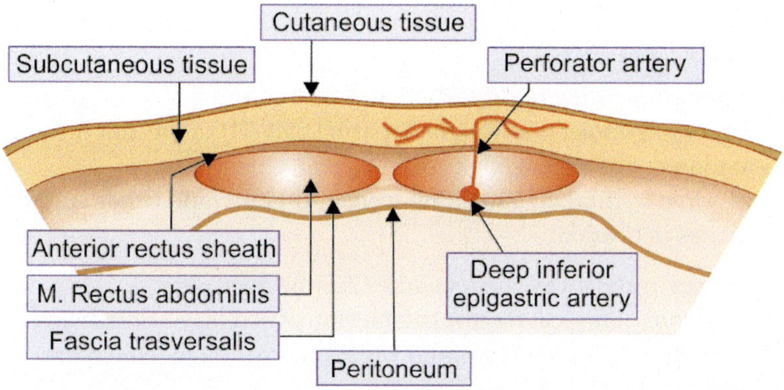

Fig. 3: Lacerations of the extra-abdominal arteries or veins, such as the inferior epigastric vessels, can result in a rectus abdominis sheath hematoma or a subfascial hematoma.
Source: Figures Taken from https://www.researchgate.net/publication/335995785/figure/fig2/AS:806648251695104@1569331338040/Extra-abdominals-arteries-or-vein-inferior-epigastric-vessels-lacerations-can-lead-to_W640.jpg.

- *Rectus sheath hematoma* ***(Fig. 3)****:* Though rare, this type can result in severe outcomes, including hypovolemic shock or consumptive coagulopathy, which may require surgical intervention.

Importance of Hemostasis

Ensuring effective hemostasis during the procedure is crucial to prevent these complications and ensure a smooth recovery for the patient. Close monitoring for signs of hematoma formation is essential in the postoperative period to address any issues promptly.

VENOUS THROMBOEMBOLISM

Pulmonary embolism is a life-threatening complication that can arise from deep venous thrombosis (DVT). The clinical presentation of PE varies based on the size of the clot and can range from mild symptoms to severe respiratory distress or cardiovascular collapse.

Diagnosis of PE is typically confirmed through:

- *Spiral CT scan:* This is the most common and effective method for diagnosing PE.
- *Pulmonary arteriography:* Considered the gold standard but less commonly used due to its invasive nature.
- *Ventilation-perfusion (V/Q) scan:* Useful, especially when CT is contraindicated.
- *Venous Doppler ultrasound:* It should be performed on the lower limbs to exclude the presence of DVT.

Treatment

Management of PE includes:

- *Therapeutic anticoagulation:* Using either unfractionated heparin (UFH) or low-molecular-weight heparin (LMWH) to prevent further clot formation.
- *Supportive treatment:* Providing oxygen therapy and other supportive measures as needed.

In some cases, more invasive procedures may be necessary:

- *Embolectomy:* Surgical removal of the clot, which may be lifesaving.
- *Thrombolysis:* The use of thrombolytic agents to dissolve clots, particularly in severe cases.

FOREIGN BODY

Retained surgical sponges and instruments after caesarean sections, though infrequent, pose significant risks, and are a major source of lawsuits and medical malpractice claims. A review of medical records related to these claims revealed that:

- Sponges account for 69% of cases.
- Instruments account for 31% of cases.

Risk Factors

The likelihood of retaining a foreign body is significantly higher in:

- Emergency surgeries
- Patients with a higher body mass index (BMI)

In one study, a falsely accurate sponge count was documented in 76% of claim cases following abdominal procedures.

Recommendations

To mitigate this risk, surgeons should routinely—explore the abdominal cavity before closure, rather than solely relying on reported sponge counts. This practice is crucial for ensuring patient safety and preventing potential complications associated with retained surgical items.

REFERENCES

1. Jadon A. Complications of regional and general anaesthesia in obstetric practice. Indian J Anaesth. 2010;54(5):415.
2. Bergholt T, Stenderup JK, Vedsted-Jakobsen A, Helm P, Lenstrup C. Intraoperative surgical complication during cesarean section: an observational study of the incidence and risk factors. Acta Obstet Gynecol Scand. 2003;82(3):251-6.
3. Mousa HA, Blum J, Abou El Senoun G, Shakur H, Alfirevic Z. Treatment for primary postpartum haemorrhage. Cochrane Pregnancy and Childbirth Group, editor. Cochrane Database Syst Rev. 2014;2017(9):CD003249.

4. Parisio-Poldiak N, Morel E, Hua C, Gibbs SL, Billue D. Cesarean Section Complications Followed by Bladder Cystotomy and Gross Hematuria Due to Unknown Dense Scar Tissue. Cureus. 2020;12(12):e11902. A
5. Zlakishvili B, Sela HY, Tankel J, Ioscovich A, Rotem R, Grisaru-Granovsky S, et al. Post-cesarean ileus: an assessment of incidence, risk factors and outcomes. Eur J Obstet Gynecol Reprod Biol. 2022;269:55-61.

8 CHAPTER

Management of Previous Caesarean Section

INTRODUCTION

The number of patients with previous caesarean section have increased. It is an ongoing challenge to decide whether trial of labor after caesarean is better than elective repeat caesarean section. This decision depends on many factors, and should be tailored to each patients needs, with the involvement of a consultant obstetrician.

REPEAT CAESAREAN SECTION

It was a popular belief that "once a caesarean always a caesarean," partly because the operation was done mainly for disproportion, and subsequent babies being usually larger, if a patient was previously incapable of delivering herself with an intact uterus, it was unlikely to expect her to deliver with a scarred uterus. Many primigravid trials of labor, however, fail because of uterine inertia or because of a persistent occiput posterior position, or malpresentation, rather than disproportion. Under favorable circumstances, therefore, a repeat caesarean section may not be necessary. Nevertheless, a previous caesarean section certainly casts "a shadow over any future pregnancy" and increases the risk of caesarean section.

Rupture of the lower segment scar is much less common compared to the upper segment caesarean. Factors that are commonly associated with subsequent scar rupture are infection of the scar and implantation of the placenta over the site of the old scar. The classical scar is more likely to rupture probably because, unlike the lower segment, the upper segment is undergoing constant and rhythmic activity in the form of 'after pains' during the early days of the puerperium, thus interfering with good healing.

A repeat caesarean section is chiefly indicated in cases of established disproportion, and a history of puerperal sepsis after the previous caesarean and after a classical caesarean section. The fact that a patient had a caesarean section before is no excuse for inflicting this surgical insult a second time. The technique of repeat caesarean section does not differ from the standard lower segment operation, except in a few details. The parietal peritoneum ought to be opened as high as possible and with great care because the bladder may be displaced upwards and the intestines may be adherent to the original wound. The ureterovesical fold is usually much shallower than in the fresh case. Extra-care should be taken in reflecting down the bladder from the lower segment, because it may be adherent and thus more liable to injury. It is safer to dissect this down by sharp dissection in the proper plane than by blunt dissection.

VAGINAL BIRTH AFTER CAESAREAN SECTION

The primary concern for women considering subsequent pregnancies after a caesarean section is the risk of uterine scar rupture. However, the increased risk is relatively small, particularly after a single lower-segment caesarean section. In a large cohort study conducted from 1999 to 2002 involving over 17,000 women attempting a trial of labor and >15,000 undergoing elective repeat caesarean sections.[1]

There was no significant difference in the rates of hysterectomy or maternal death between the two groups.

The risk of rupture varies based on the type of previous uterine incision:
- *Classical or T-shaped scars:* 4–9%
- *Low vertical incisions:* 1–7%
- *Low transverse incisions:* 0.2–1.5%

Vaginal Birth after Caesarean Success Rates

Success rates for vaginal birth after caesarean (VBAC) range from 60 to 80%. However, maternal and neonatal morbidity in women attempting VBAC is often linked to cases where VBAC is unsuccessful.

Factors Influencing Vaginal Birth after Caesarean Success

Careful patient selection is crucial for maximizing the chances of a successful VBAC. Factors associated with unsuccessful VBAC include:
- Induced labor
- Previous caesarean for the arrest of labor
- Advanced maternal age
- High maternal body mass index (BMI)
- High birth weight
- Shorter interdelivery interval

Overall, while the risks associated with VBAC are low, thorough assessment and appropriate.

Who Should Be Offered Vaginal Birth after Caesarean Section?

Women at a gestational age of 37–40 weeks with a previous lower segment caesarean section performed for a non-recurring indication can be offered a trial of labor (TOL) if there are no contraindications to vaginal delivery. This includes women with:
- Two previous low transverse scars who have had a vaginal delivery in the past.
- Low vertical scars, as TOL is also permissible in these cases.

Important Considerations

- *Pelvic adequacy:* The pelvis must be assessed to ensure it is adequate for vaginal delivery.
- *Placenta location:* It is crucial to evaluate the placenta's position. If it is low-lying and anterior, there is a risk of placenta accreta. Ultrasound with color Doppler can help identify this condition. A low-lying placenta is a contraindication for TOL due to the risk of morbid adherence.

Setting for Vaginal Birth after Caesarean Section

Vaginal birth after caesarean should only be attempted in a facility equipped for an immediate caesarean section, with experienced obstetricians and anesthetists available 24/7. Access to blood transfusion services is also essential.

Contraindications to Vaginal Birth after Caesarean

- Previous classical or inverted T-shaped uterine incision
- History of uterine rupture (the risk of repeat rupture is significantly higher with a classical incision: 6% with a lower segment scar versus 32% with an upper segment scar)
- Contracted pelvis
- Medical or obstetric complications that prevent safe vaginal birth (e.g., placenta previa).

By carefully evaluating these factors, healthcare providers can better ensure the safety and success of VBAC for eligible women.

INDUCTION OF VAGINAL BIRTH AFTER CAESAREAN SECTION

Induction of labor is not contraindicated for women contemplating VBAC, although spontaneous labor is associated with a higher success rate. Here are key points regarding induction methods:

- *Induction methods and uterine rupture risks*
    - *Oxytocin:* Generally considered safer for inducing labor in women with a history of caesarean section. A study reported a uterine rupture rate of 1.1% with oxytocin use.[2]
    - *Prostaglandins:* The use of prostaglandins, particularly misoprostol, is contraindicated in women with a previous caesarean due to higher risks.
    - *Dinoprostone:* Associated with a rupture rate of 2%.
    - *Misoprostol:* Linked to a significantly higher rupture rate of 6%.
- *General findings:* A population-based study indicated that uterine rupture rates were:
    - 0.52% with spontaneous labor
    - 0.77% with induced labor (without prostaglandins)
    - 2.45% with prostaglandin-induced labor.

AMERICAN COLLEGE OF OBSTETRICIANS AND GYNECOLOGISTS RECOMMENDATIONS

The ACOG Committee on Obstetric Practice Emphasizes:[3] The risk of uterine rupture is increased with any induction method, but the absolute risk remains low. Sequential use of prostaglandins and oxytocin should be avoided. Misoprostol should not be used in women with a previous caesarean or uterine surgery.

In summary, while induction can be performed in VBAC candidates, careful selection of induction agents and methods is essential to minimize risks.

INDUCTION OF LABOR FOR VAGINAL BIRTH AFTER CAESAREAN SECTION

Women attempting VBAC require vigilant monitoring by experienced healthcare staff who can recognize the signs of imminent uterine rupture. Key monitoring parameters include:

- *Maternal vital signs:* Frequent checks of pulse and blood pressure.
- *Uterine contractions:* Regular assessment of contraction patterns.
- *Fetal heart rate:* Continuous electronic fetal monitoring is recommended when facilities are available, as nonreassuring fetal heart rate patterns may indicate uterine rupture.

Signs of Uterine Rupture

- *Fetal bradycardia:* Often the most consistent finding associated with uterine rupture.
- *Suprapubic pain and tenderness:* Pain may occur, though tenderness can also be present in a nonscarred uterus.
- *Loss of station of presenting part:* Notable changes in fetal positioning.
- *Vaginal bleeding:* Any unusual bleeding should be investigated.
- *Signs of hypovolemia:* Indications of significant blood loss.

Pain Management

Epidural analgesia: Not contraindicated in VBAC, providing effective pain relief without increasing rupture risk.

External Cephalic Version

Breech presentation: External cephalic version can be successfully performed in women with a previous caesarean section, similar to those without prior surgeries.

In summary, thorough monitoring and appropriate pain management strategies are essential for ensuring the safety of women attempting VBAC.

REFERENCES

1. Landon MB, Grobman WA; Eunice Kennedy Shriver National Institute of Child Health and Human Development Maternal-Fetal Medicine Units Network. What We Have Learned About Trial of Labor After Cesarean Delivery from the Maternal-Fetal Medicine Units Cesarean Registry. Semin Perinatol. 2016;40(5):281-6.
2. Ophir E, Odeh M, Hirsch Y, Bornstein J. Uterine rupture during trial of labor: controversy of induction's methods. Obstet Gynecol Surv. 2012;67(11):734-45.
3. ACOG Practice Bulletin No. 205: Vaginal Birth After Cesarean Delivery. Obstet Gynecol. 2019;133(2):e110-27.

9

CHAPTER

Enhanced Recovery after Caesarean Birth

INTRODUCTION

Enhanced recovery after surgery (ERAS) is a standardized perioperative care program designed to improve patient outcomes and optimize healthcare resources based on scientific evidence. The ERAS Society has developed a specific pathway for caesarean birth that encompasses the entire perioperative process, from the decision to operate to hospital discharge.

Key components of the ERAS pathway for caesarean birth:[1]

- Preoperative preparation
- *Patient education:* Informing patients about the procedure, recovery expectations, and discharge planning.
- *Nutritional optimization:* Encouraging patients to maintain adequate nutrition before surgery.
- *Preoperative assessment:* Evaluating medical history and potential risk factors.

PERIOPERATIVE CARE

- *Minimizing fasting:* Allowing clear fluids up to 2 hours before surgery.
- *Multimodal analgesia:* Using a combination of analgesic techniques to manage pain effectively and reduce opioid use.
- *Antibiotic prophylaxis:* Administering prophylactic antibiotics to reduce the risk of infection.

INTRAOPERATIVE MANAGEMENT

Fluid management careful management of intravenous fluids to prevent overhydration or dehydration.

Minimally invasive techniques: Where appropriate, using techniques that minimize tissue trauma.

POSTOPERATIVE MONITORING

- *Early mobilization:* Encouraging patients to get out of bed and move soon after surgery.
- *Nutritional support:* Initiating early oral intake as tolerated.
    - Discharge planning preparing for discharge as early as possible, focusing on the patient's recovery and support at home.

  - Immediate neonatal care. Ensuring optimal care for the newborn immediately after birth, including skin-to-skin contact and early breastfeeding.

Benefits:

- Implementing the ERAS pathway for caesarean births has been shown to:
  - Improve patient recovery times.
  - Reduce hospital stays.
- Lower complication rates.
- Enhance overall patient satisfaction.

By following this evidence-based approach, healthcare providers can significantly improve outcomes for both mothers and their newborns.

REFERENCE

1. Ubom EO, Wang C, Klocksieben F, Flicker AB, Diven L, Rochon M, et al. Enhanced recovery protocol after cesarean delivery: impact on opioid use and pain perception. AJOG Glob Rep. 2023;3(3):100220.

CHAPTER

10 Concurrent Surgeries with Caesarean Section

INTRODUCTION

Surgeries like tubal ligation, caesarean myomectomy and caesarean hysterectomy, in cases of placenta accreta spectrum or as a last resort, in postpartum hemorrhage, can be done concurrently with a caesarean section.

STERILIZATION

During a second caesarean section, it is important to discuss the option of sterilization with the patient, especially if she has a healthy child and does not wish to have more children. Here are the key points for counseling and procedure:

COUNSELING POINTS

- *Fertility considerations:* Explain that sterilization is a permanent method of contraception.
- *Written consent:* Ensure both partners provide informed written consent prior to the procedure.

SURGICAL TECHNIQUE[1] (FIGS. 1A TO D)

- *Modified Pomeroy technique:* This is the preferred method for sterilization during caesarean sections.
- *Identification of the fallopian tubes:* The uterus is gently displaced to one side to access the tubes.
- *Loop formation:* A loop of the tube is formed approximately 3 cm from the cornual end and secured with absorbable catgut sutures.
- *Tubal segment excision:* The tied segment of the tube is excised and sent for histopathological examination.

POSTOPERATIVE CONSIDERATIONS

Absorbable sutures: Using absorbable sutures helps to minimize the risk of recanalization by allowing the ends of the tube to separate over time.

By discussing these aspects thoroughly, patients can make informed decisions about their reproductive health.

CAESAREAN MYOMECTOMY AND HYSTERECTOMY

Caesarean Myomectomy[2]

Myomectomy during a caesarean section has traditionally been viewed as a high-risk procedure due to the increased vascularity of the uterus, which

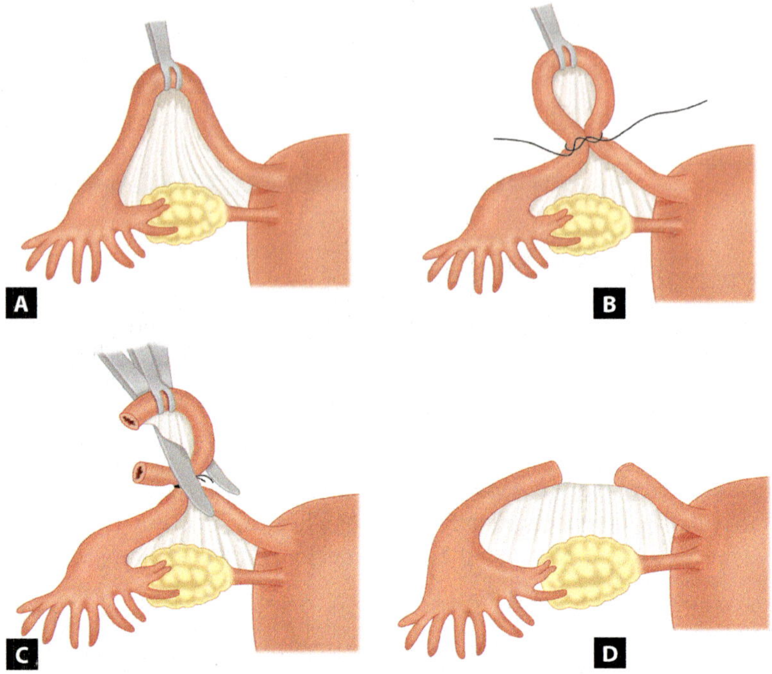

Figs. 1A to D: Pomeroy or modified Pomeroy technique. (A) A loop of the proximal tubal ampulla is elevated, exposing the vascular supply of the mesosalpinx; (B) An absorbable suture is used to ligate the loop bilaterally, ensuring both tubal occlusion and hemostasis; (C) A hemostat is applied to the suture strands just distal to the knot to prevent the tube from retracting into the abdomen. Using the open blade of Metzenbaum scissors, the mesosalpinx is pierced, and approximately 1 cm of the tube is excised; and (D) As the absorbable suture material dissolves, the proximal and distal portions of the tube return to their original positions, ensuring tubal interruption.
Source: https://resources.ama.uk.com/glowm_www/graphics/figures/v6/0390/001f.gif

raises concerns about the risk of sutures cutting through. However, the key consideration is the necessity of the myomectomy itself.

Indications for Myomectomy

- *Unnecessary procedures:* Many myomectomies performed during caesarean sections may not be warranted. It is often advisable to reassess the need for myomectomy after pregnancy, once the uterus has returned to its normal size.
- *Clear indications:* In cases where there is a clear medical necessity, recent literature supports the safety of performing myomectomy concurrently with caesarean section, provided that the patient is appropriately selected. This approach can help avoid the need for a second surgery without significantly increasing maternal morbidity.

Considerations for Safety

Safer cases: Myomectomy is generally safer for certain types of fibroids, including:

- Anterior wall myomas
- Subserous and pedunculated myomas: These can often be removed without additional incisions.

Higher risk cases: More complex situations, such as multiple myomas.

Deep intramural, fundal, cornual, and posterior wall myomas: These may lead to greater surgical complications and are better addressed with an interval myomectomy instead.

CAESAREAN HYSTERECTOMY

The incidence of peripartum hysterectomy, encompassing both caesarean and postpartum hysterectomies, ranges from 0.25 to 0.8 per 1,000 deliveries.[3] This risk is significantly elevated after a caesarean section—up to 5–10 times greater compared to vaginal births.

Common Indications

- *Intractable uterine hemorrhage:* This is the leading cause for performing a caesarean hysterectomy, particularly when bleeding cannot be controlled through conservative measures.
- *Placenta accreta:* This condition, especially when associated with placenta previa, often necessitates a hysterectomy.
- *Uterine rupture:* Emergency situations may require rapid intervention.

Surgical Considerations

- *Procedure steps:* The principles of a caesarean hysterectomy are similar to those of an abdominal hysterectomy. Quick closure of the uterine incision is crucial to minimize blood loss.
- *Uterine exteriorization:* This is typically performed, and the uterus is placed under tension to facilitate the procedure.
- *Challenges:* Edematous pelvic tissues and lax broad ligaments can complicate the surgery, increasing the risk of ureteral injury due to more lateral clamping of the broad ligaments.

Hysterectomy Types

- *Subtotal hysterectomy:* Often performed in cases of ongoing hemorrhage to achieve rapid control of bleeding.
- *Total hysterectomy:* Indicated when there is a cervical tear or significant bleeding from placenta previa. However, distinguishing between total and subtotal hysterectomy can be challenging if the cervix is not clearly identifiable during surgery.

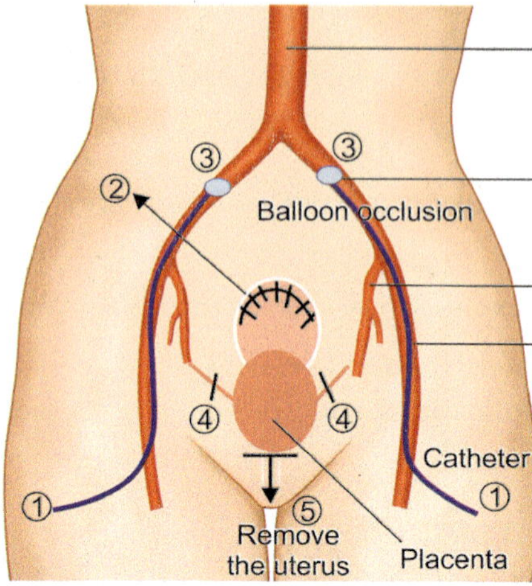

Fig. 2: Anatomy in the pelvis and caesarean hysterectomy procedure.
Source: https://www.researchgate.net/profile/Masafumi-Koshiyama/publication/313260834/figure/fig1/AS:457865413566465@1486175029974/Anatomy-in-the-Pelvis-and-Cesarean-Hysterectomy-Procedure-For-more-Information-see-the_W640.jpg

Figure 2 shows the anatomic considerations while performing caesarean hysterectomy.

The procedure carries a high risk of complications, including:

- Urinary tract injury
- Relaparotomy
- Massive transfusion
- Disseminated intravascular coagulopathy

A case fatality rate of approximately 4% has been reported, emphasizing the serious nature of emergency hysterectomy.

Indications

Beyond obstetric emergencies, gynaecological reasons for performing a hysterectomy post-caesarean are limited. Although some may consider hysterectomy for benign conditions (e.g., fibroids), the ability to carry a pregnancy to term typically suggests that these conditions do not warrant surgical intervention.

This information highlights the critical need for careful evaluation and management of patients who may require peripartum hysterectomy, balancing the risks and benefits involved.

REFERENCES

1. Schmidt EO, Diedrich JT, Eisenberg DL. (2014). Surgical procedures for tubal sterilization. Glob Libr Womens Med. [Online] Available from https://www.glowm.com/section-view/item/399 [Last accessed December, 2024].

2. Goyal M, Dawood AS, Elbohoty SB, Abbas AM, Singh P, Melana N, et al. Cesarean myomectomy in the last ten years; A true shift from contraindication to indication: a systematic review and meta-analysis. Eur J Obstet Gynecol Reprod Biol. 2021;256:145-57.
3. Kwee A, Bots ML, Visser GHA, Bruinse HW. Emergency peripartum hysterectomy: a prospective study in The Netherlands. Eur J Obstet Gynecol Reprod Biol. 2006;124(2):187-92.

CHAPTER 11

Optimizing Caesarean Sections

INTRODUCTION

Optimizing caesarean sections (CSs) is crucial for improving maternal and neonatal outcomes, reducing unnecessary interventions, and ensuring that the procedure is used only when medically necessary.

GLOBAL EPIDEMIOLOGY OF CAESAREAN SECTION USAGE AND DISPARITIES

For mothers and newborns experiencing problems such as antepartum hemorrhage, fetal distress, atypical fetal presentation, and hypertensive disorders, CS is an essential life-saving treatment. In many nations, it is now the most common major operation performed.[1] CS rates have increased dramatically during the last 30 years, exceeding the 10–15% of births that are thought to be ideal. In many middle- and high-income nations, nonmedically indicated CS is the primary cause of this rise. On the other hand, no data suggests that CS rates higher than 20% enhance prenatal or neonatal outcomes on a population level. On the other hand, CS rates are still below 10% in many low- and middle-income nations, indicating restricted availability of this necessary procedure.

Within low- and middle-income countries, there are notable differences in the CS between the wealthiest and poorest populations. Even though CS can save lives, its widespread use—especially for nonmedical purposes—is troubling because of the risks it poses to expectant mothers and their babies. In 2015, more over 50% of live deliveries globally were delivered through CS, with rates higher than those supported by obstetric needs in the majority of nations. While insufficient access to healthcare is still a major problem in low-income and some middle-income nations, particularly among the poorest women, wealthier women and private healthcare facilities frequently exhibit notably high rates of CS.

This underuse of CS puts women and babies at greater risk of death due to the lack of access to life-saving surgical care during childbirth. There is an urgent need to optimize CS usage, driven by a deeper understanding of the factors influencing its overuse and a concerted effort to ensure universal access for all women. CS is one of the few medical interventions with such global and regional disparities in use.

SHORT- AND LONG-TERM EFFECTS OF CAESAREAN SECTION ON THE HEALTH OF WOMEN AND CHILDREN

Short- and Long-term Effects of Caesarean Section on Women's Health

- *Severe acute maternal morbidity (SAMM)*—has been used as a proxy measure for maternal death, with several definitions. It refers to the occurrence of complications such as hemorrhage requiring hysterectomy or blood transfusion, any hysterectomy, uterine rupture, anesthetic-related complications (arising from the use of general or local anesthesia, analgesics, or other sedation during labor and delivery), obstetric shock, cardiac arrest, acute renal failure, assisted ventilation or intubation, puerperal venous thromboembolism, major puerperal infections, wound disruption in the hospital, and hematoma. Large population-based studies consistently show that the unadjusted frequency of severe acute maternal morbidity is higher following CS compared to vaginal birth.
- *Short-term and long-term morbidity:* Long-term sequelae of CS include pelvic adhesions, small bowel obstruction, menorrhagia, dysmenorrhea, and chronic pain.
- *Maternal mortality:* The absolute risk of maternal death associated with CS is known to be low in high-resource settings, and higher in low-resource settings.[2] Scheduled CSs pose a lower mortality risk compared to emergency CS performed during labor. While maternal death is uncommon, studies indicate that the risk of death from an emergency intrapartum CS can be up to four times greater than with vaginal delivery.[3] Moreover, the likelihood of maternal death during childbirth increases in subsequent pregnancies after a previous CS, due to a higher risk of uterine rupture and abnormal placentation.
- *Adverse outcomes for women in subsequent pregnancy:* Following a CS, future pregnancies carry heightened risks of hysterectomy, abnormal placentation, uterine rupture, stillbirth, and preterm birth.[4] As the number of CSs increases, there is also a greater likelihood of complications such as excessive bleeding, the need for blood transfusions, adhesions, intraoperative surgical injuries, and hysterectomy.

Short- and Long-term Outcomes for Infants and Children

Intrauterine Effects on Infant Health

Intrauterine exposures significantly impact an infant's lifelong health. Emerging evidence suggests that the birth process and interventions during labor can also influence normal physiological or pathophysiological development. Babies delivered by CS experience different hormonal, physical, bacterial, and medical interventions, including intrapartum antibiotics and uterotonics, which may subtly alter their physiology. Additionally, many planned CSs are performed before 39 weeks of gestation, which may increase the risk of respiratory issues and hypoglycemia in newborns.

INTERVENTIONS TO REDUCE UNNECESSARY CAESAREAN SECTIONS IN HEALTHY WOMEN AND BABIES

Interventions to reduce unnecessary CSs can be broadly classified as clinical and nonclinical, although there is an overlap between the two.

Clinical Interventions

Only two clinical interventions for healthy women and babies with no complications.

1. Effectiveness of routine induction of labor at or near term.
2. Active management of labor.

In an attempt to reduce the incidence of CS at LTMGH and Sion Hospital, a tertiary referral center for complex obstetric cases, Dr Niranjan N Chavan devised a "Sion Model" in July 2023 that has reduced C-sections by 10% in the last year. A study of 345 pregnant women showed counseling and patient education are key to promoting vaginal birth. "Reducing C-section rates is crucial in improving maternal and neonatal health." Approximately 1,500–1,700 deliveries annually occur in Sion Hospital.

What is the Sion Model?

Sion model method: Revolutionizing labor induction—the Sion Model, a *novel approach to labor induction*, has significantly impacted CS rates **(Fig. 1)**.

This model *leverages mechanical dilatation methods, specifically, Foley's catheter (24 Fr) and dinoprostone gel (250–500 μg) combination*, to effectively dilate and open the cervix followed by augmentation of labor leads to vaginal birth.

CRITERIAS FOR SION MODEL

Inclusion Criteria

Singleton full-term cephalic pregnancy:

- Primigravida
- Multigravida
- Previous one LSCS patients

Exclusion Criteria

- Contraindications for vaginal delivery cephalopelvic disproportion, contracted pelvis.
- Breech presentation and all malpresentation.
- Factors warranting an elective repeat caesarean such as the previous two LSCS, previous classical caesarean, hysterotomy, and myomectomy.

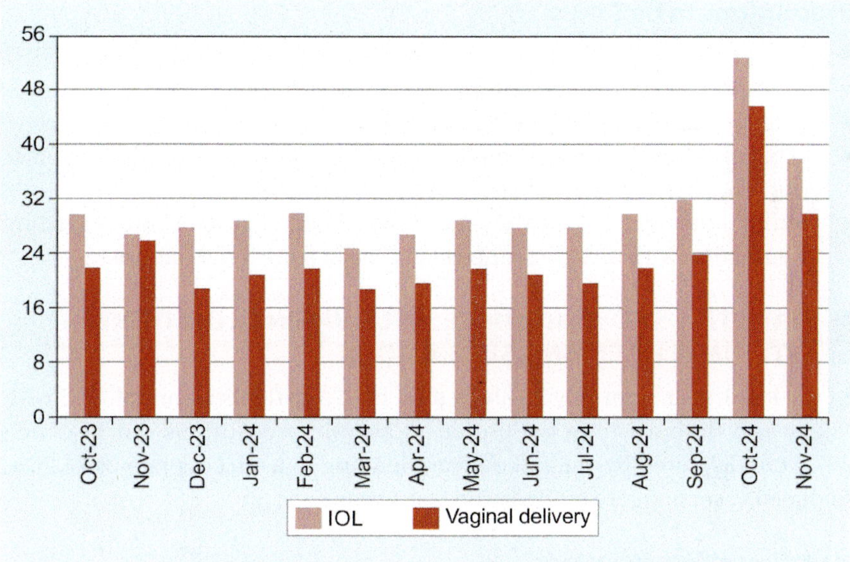

Month	*IOL with Foley's and dinoprostone gel*	*Vaginal delivery*	*Success rate (%)*
July 23	32	24	75
Aug 23	31	25	80
Sept 23	29	20	69
Oct 23	30	22	73
Nov 23	27	22	81
Dec 23	28	19	67
Jan 24	29	21	72
Feb 24	30	22	73
Mar 24	25	19	76
April 24	27	20	74
May 24	29	22	76
June 24	28	21	75
July 24	28	20	71
Aug 24	30	22	73
Sept 24	32	24	75
Oct 24	53	46	86
Nov 24	38	30	78.6
Total	526	399	75.8

Fig. 1: Statistics showing successful vaginal delivery after implementing the Sion model. (IOL: induction of labor)

Precautions to be Taken

- Offer labor analgesia.
- Monitor for uterine hyperstimulation and abruption.
- Intrapartum fetal heart rate monitoring.
- In patients with scarred uterus, monitor signs of scar dehiscence such as scar tenderness, maternal tachycardia, and fetal bradycardia.
- Senior obstetrician opinion recommended for a decision regarding reinduction with dinoprostone gel in case of a previous caesarean.

STATISTICS SHOWING SUCCESSFUL VAGINAL DELIVERY AFTER IMPLEMENTING SION MODEL

In the last 1 year from July 23–24, a total of 373 patients were induced with foleys and dinoprostone gel under all aseptic precautions out of which 277 were delivered by vaginal delivery leading to a success rate of 74.26%. Reduced C-section rate by 7% in the last 1 year.

Nonclinical Interventions

- *Interventions targeted at women, families, and communities:* Factors such as fear, safety concerns, convenience, misinformation, and societal or peer-group norms play a significant role in shaping women's and their families' decisions regarding the mode of birth. Most women reported that face-to-face discussions with healthcare professionals had a strong influence on their decision-making, especially when clinicians acknowledged childbirth as an emotional experience rather than purely a medical procedure. However, frustration and mistrust arose when women felt their concerns were not heard or when the advice given was inconsistent.
- *Interventions targeted at health professionals:* Health professionals' use of CSs is influenced by concerns about litigation, peer and organizational norms, financial incentives, and convenience. Efforts to optimize CS use among healthcare providers have included educational programs to promote adherence to evidence-based practices, second-opinion policies, audits with feedback, and peer reviews of CS indications.[5] Two interventions that showed a slight reduction in CS rates involved the implementation of evidence-based guidelines alongside mandatory second opinions and the use of evidence-based guidelines combined with CS audits and timely feedback.

CONCLUSION

- *Clear guidelines and protocols:* Establishing standardized clinical guidelines helps healthcare providers make informed decisions, minimizing elective or nonmedically indicated C-sections.

- *Enhanced prenatal care:* Early identification and management of pregnancy complications can reduce the need for emergency C-sections, allowing more time to plan for potential vaginal deliveries were safe.
- *Promoting vaginal birth after caesarean (VBAC):* Encouraging and safely managing VBAC for eligible women helps reduce repeat C-sections, lowering associated risks with multiple surgeries.
- *Adequate labor support:* Providing comprehensive labor support, including access to skilled birth attendants, continuous monitoring, and appropriate pain relief, can help avoid unnecessary C-sections by facilitating vaginal delivery.
- *Reducing fear of litigation:* Addressing the fear of legal consequences in obstetric care can prevent the overuse of C-sections, promoting evidence-based decision-making.
- By implementing these strategies, healthcare systems can optimize the use of CS, ensuring they are performed safely when indicated and reducing potential complications associated with overuse. This approach leads to better health outcomes for both mothers and babies, while also addressing healthcare costs and resource allocation.

REFERENCES

1. Khatamee M. Historical perspective "Rostam" is born: how? By Cesarean section (940–1020?). ACOG Clin Rev. 2000;(2):12.
2. Hawkins JL, Koonin LM, Palmer SK, Gibbs CP. Anesthesia-related Deaths during Obstetric Delivery in the United States, 1979–1990. Anesthesiology. 1997;86(2):277-84.
3. Mathai M, Hofmeyr GJ, Mathai NE. Abdominal surgical incisions for caesarean section. Cochrane Pregnancy and Childbirth Group, editor. Cochrane Database Syst Rev [Internet]. 2013 May 31 [cited 2024 Dec 24];2013(5). Available from: http://doi.wiley.com/10.1002/14651858.CD004453.pub3
4. Hohlagschwandtner M. Is the formation of a bladder flap at cesarean necessary? A randomized trial. Obstet Gynecol. 2001;98(6):1089-92.
5. Ophir E, Odeh M, Hirsch Y, Bornstein J. Uterine Rupture During Trial of Labor: Controversy of Induction's Methods. Obstet Gynecol Surv. 2012;67(11):734-45.

12 CHAPTER Multiple Choice Questions

1. **The primary benefit of using a low segment transverse incision for caesarean delivery as opposed to a classical incision is:**
   a. Reduced blood loss
   b. Lower risk of uterine rupture in future pregnancies
   c. Easier access to the uterine cavity
   d. Faster recovery time

Ans. b. Lower risk of uterine rupture in future pregnancies

2. **In a patient who is undergoing a planned caesarean section at term, which of the following should be routinely administered preoperatively?**
   a. Intravenous antibiotics
   b. Anticoagulants for deep vein thrombosis prophylaxis
   c. Prophylactic tocolytics
   d. Epidural anesthesia for pain management

Ans. a. Intravenous antibiotics

3. **After a caesarean section, the most common cause of postpartum hemorrhage (PPH) is:**
   a. Uterine atony
   b. Genital tract lacerations
   c. Placenta accreta
   d. Retained products of conception

Ans. a. Uterine atony

4. **The risk of uterine rupture during labor is lowest if:**
   a. She has a history of vaginal delivery
   b. There is an interval of at least 2 years between pregnancies
   c. She is induced with prostaglandins
   d. The caesarean section was performed for fetal distress

Ans. b. There is an interval of at least 2 years between pregnancies

5. **According to the American College of Obstetricians and Gynecologists (ACOG), the most important factor in deciding whether to attempt a vaginal birth after caesarean (VBAC) is:**
   a. The type of previous caesarean scar
   b. The maternal age
   c. The presence of a favorable cervix
   d. The parity of the patient

Ans. a. The type of previous caesarean scar

6. According to Robsons classification, previous caesarean section, single cephalic pregnancy, at least 37 weeks' gestation would come under group?

a. 2
b. 3
c. 4
d. 5

Ans. d. 5

7. Risk of fetal laceration at caesarean delivery is:

a. 10%
b. 2%
c. 20%
d. 5%

Ans. b. 2%

8. Pfannenstiel incision would be described as:

a. 2 cm above pubic symphysis, transverse, curved
b. 5 cm above pubic symphysis, transverse, straight
c. Vertical incision
d. Muscle cutting incision

Ans. a. 2 cm above pubic symphysis, transverse, curved

9. Closure of parietal peritoneum during caesarean section is associated with:

a. More postoperative pain
b. Infection
c. More hemorrhage
d. Doesn't change postoperative course

Ans. a. More postoperative pain

Index

Page numbers followed by *f* refer to figure and *t* refer to table.